P9-BUI-674

Contents

The Shopper's Guide to GI Values

The Authoritative Source of Glycemic Index Values for More Than 1,200 Foods

Dr. Jennie Brand-Miller
and Kaye Foster-Powell
with Fiona Atkinson

Da Capo
∞
LIFE
LONG

A MEMBER OF THE
PERSEUS BOOKS GROUP

Other Titles in the New Glucose Revolution Series

For the definitive overview of the glycemic index . . .

> *The Low GI Handbook: The New Glucose Revolution Guide to the Long-term Health Benefits of Low GI Eating*

For a focus on recipes, shopping, and the GI in the larger nutrition picture . . .

> *The New Glucose Revolution Low GI Vegetarian Cookbook*

For a basic introduction to the GI plus the top 100 low GI foods . . .

> *The New Glucose Revolution Low GI Eating Made Easy: The Beginner's Guide to Eating with the Glycemic Index*

For a focus on weight loss . . .

> *The Low GI Diet Revolution: The Definitive Science-Based Weight Loss Plan*

> *The New Glucose Revolution Low GI Guide to Losing Weight: The Only Authoritative Guide to Weight Loss Using the Glycemic Index*

For a focus on the GI and specific health conditions . . .

> *Everything You Need to Know to Manage Type 2 Diabetes: Simple Steps for Surviving and Thriving with the Low GI Plan*

> *The New Glucose Revolution Low GI Gluten-Free Eating Made Easy: The Essential Guide to the Glycemic Index and Gluten-Free Living*

> *The New Glucose Revolution Low GI Guide to the Metabolic Syndrome and Your Heart: The Only Authoritative Guide to Using the Glycemic Index for Better Heart Health*

> *The New Glucose Revolution What Makes My Blood Glucose Go Up . . . And Down?: 101 Frequently Asked Questions about Your Blood Glucose Level*

> *The Low GI Guide to Living Well with PCOS: Lose Weight, Boost Fertility, and Gain Control over Polycystic Ovarian Syndrome with the Glycemic Index*

To stay up to date with the latest research on carbohydrates, the GI, and your health, and the latest books in the series, check out the free online monthly newsletter *GI News*, produced by Dr. Jennie Brand-Miller's GI Group at the University of Sydney: http://ginews.blogspot.com

About the authors

Jennie Brand-Miller, Ph.D., one of the world's foremost authorities on carbohydrates and the glycemic index, has championed the GI approach to nutrition for more than 25 years. Professor of Nutrition at the University of Sydney and past president of the Nutrition Society of Australia, in 2004 Brand-Miller was awarded Australia's prestigious ATSE Clunies Ross Award for her commitment to advancing science and technology. She is an in-demand speaker at scientific conferences, and her laboratory at the University of Sydney is one of the world's busiest GI-testing centers. Professor Brand-Miller is coauthor of the more than fifteen books in the internationally bestselling *New Glucose Revolution* series, which has more than 3.5 million copies in print worldwide.

Kaye Foster-Powell, BSc., M. Nutr. & Diet., an accredited practicing dietitian with extensive experience in diabetes management, is the coauthor, with Dr. Brand-Miller and Fiona Atkinson, of the authoritative tables of GI and glycemic load values published in *Diabetes Care*. Foster-Powell is also coauthor with Brand-Miller of the more than fifteen books in the internationally bestselling *New Glucose Revolution* series.

Fiona Atkinson, BSc., M. Nutr. & Diet., is a research dietitian and the manager of the University of Sydney's Glycemic Index Research Service (SUGiRS). Along with Jennie Brand-Miller and Kaye Foster-Powell, she is the author of the authoritative tables of GI and glycemic load values published in *Diabetes Care*. She is pursuing a Ph.D. at the University of Sydney focusing on the glycemic index.

OPM

10 9 8 7 6 5 4 3 2

10 steps to a healthy low GI life for everybody, every day, every meal

- ❏ Eat seven or more servings of fruit and vegetables every day
- ❏ Eat low GI breads and cereals, especially whole-grain versions
- ❏ Eat more legumes including soybeans, chickpeas, and lentils
- ❏ Eat small portions of nuts regularly
- ❏ Eat more fish and seafood
- ❏ Eat lean red meat, chicken, and eggs
- ❏ Eat low fat dairy foods or calcium-enriched soy products
- ❏ Avoid trans fat, eat less saturated fat, and replace with good mono- and polyunsaturates
- ❏ Limit your alcohol intake and use of salt
- ❏ Be active—don't sit for long periods. Even 30 seconds of activity will rev up your metabolism.

Understanding
the GI

Using the Shopper's Guide

We have put together this handy guide full of GI values to help you put those low GI smart carb food choices into your shopping cart and on your plate. By doing so, you'll satisfy your hunger, increase your energy levels, and eliminate your desire to eat more than you should.

Some foods that have been tested by accredited laboratories display the certified GI symbol. But what about the rest? With tables listing the GI of hundreds of foods—from breads and breakfast bars to fruit juice, fruit, and vegetables—this book will save you time in the supermarket by directing you to the best low GI foods available.

You can use the GI tables on pages 98–247 to:

❏ find the GI of your favorite foods

❏ compare foods within a category (two types of bread, for example)

❏ improve your diet by finding a low GI substitute for high GI foods

❏ put together a low GI meal

❏ shop for low GI foods including gluten-free options

The GI explained

The GI is a physiologically based measure of the effect carbohydrates have on blood glucose levels. It provides an easy and delicious way to eat a healthy diet and, at the same time, control fluctuations in blood glucose. After testing hundreds of foods around the world, scientists have now found that meals with a low GI will have less of an effect on blood glucose levels than those with a high GI.

❑ Carbohydrates that break down rapidly during digestion, releasing glucose quickly into the bloodstream, have a high GI.

❑ Carbohydrates that break down slowly, releasing glucose gradually into the bloodstream, have a low GI.

The rate of carbohydrate digestion has important implications for everybody. For most people, foods with a low GI have advantages over those with a high GI. They can:

❑ Improve blood glucose control

❑ Increase satiety, as they are more filling and satisfying and reduce appetite

❑ Facilitate weight loss

❑ Improve blood fat profiles

❑ Reduce risks of developing diabetes, heart disease, and certain types of cancer

What are the benefits of a low GI diet?

Knowing the GI values of individual foods is your key to the enormous health benefits of a low GI diet.

Low GI eating has science on its side. It's not a fad diet. There are no strict rules or regimens to follow. It's essentially about making simple adjustments to your usual eating habits—such as swapping one type of bread or breakfast cereal for another.

You'll find that you can live with it for life.

Low GI eating:

❑ Reduces swings in blood glucose
❑ Reduces your insulin levels and helps you burn fat
❑ Lowers your cholesterol levels
❑ Helps control your appetite
❑ Halves your risk of heart disease and diabetes
❑ Is suitable for your whole family
❑ Means you are eating foods closer to the way nature intended
❑ Doesn't defy common sense!

Not only that: you will feel better and have more energy—and you don't have to deprive or discipline yourself. A low GI diet is easy and has particular benefits for people who are overweight or have diabetes, hypertension, elevated blood fats, heart disease, or the metabolic syndrome (Syndrome X).

Understanding the GI of foods helps you choose the right amount of carbohydrate and the right sort of carbohydrate for your long-term health and well-being.

A low GI diet has been scientifically proven to help people:

❑ With type 1 diabetes

❑ With type 2 diabetes

❑ With gestational diabetes (diabetes during pregnancy)

❑ Who are overweight

❑ Who have lost weight and want to prevent weight re-gain

❑ Who have a normal weight but excess abdominal fat (central obesity or a potbelly)

❑ Whose blood glucose levels are higher than desirable

❑ Who have been told they have prediabetes, "impaired glucose tolerance," or a "touch of diabetes"

❑ With high levels of triglycerides and low levels of HDL cholesterol ("good" cholesterol)

❑ With metabolic syndrome (insulin resistance syndrome or Syndrome X)

❑ Who suffer from polycystic ovarian syndrome (PCOS)

❑ Who suffer from fatty liver disease (NAFLD or NASH)

If you would like to know more about the beneficial effects eating low GI foods can have on the above conditions, please refer to our other *New Glucose Revolution* books, a complete list of which is shown at the beginning of this book.

Low GI
eating

Making the change

Eating the low GI way simply involves replacing high GI foods in your diet with low GI foods. This could mean eating muesli at breakfast instead of wheat flakes, low GI bread instead of normal white or whole wheat bread, or a sparkling apple juice in place of a soft drink.

You don't need to count numbers or do any sort of mental arithmetic to make sure you are eating a healthy low GI diet.

Tips for putting the GI into practice

Be aware! Only carbohydrate-containing foods have GI values

The diet we eat contains three main nutrients: protein, carbohydrate, and fat. Some foods, such as meat, are high in protein, while bread is high in carbohydrate and butter is high in fat. We need to consume a variety of foods (in varying proportions) to provide all three nutrients, but the GI applies only to carbohydrate-rich foods. It is impossible for us to measure a GI value for foods like meat that contain negligible carbohydrate. The same applies to cheese, eggs, avocado, butter, oil, and alcohol. It is incorrect to refer to these foods as high or low GI. There are other nutritional aspects that you could consider in choosing these foods: for example, the amount and type of fats they contain.

The GI is not intended to stand alone

We don't categorize foods as "good" or "bad" according to their GI. While you will benefit from eating low GI foods at each meal, this doesn't have to be at the exclusion of all others. High GI foods like most potatoes and bread still make valuable nutritional contributions to our diet. And low GI foods like pastry that are high in saturated fat are no better for us because of their low GI. The nutritional benefits of different foods are many and varied, and it is advisable for you to base your food choices on the overall nutritional content of a food, particularly considering the saturated fat, salt, and fiber in addition to GI.

You don't need to add up the GI each day

Although we can predict the GI of a menu for the whole day, we can't predict the GI of many recipes, especially those using flour. That's why we now prefer simply to categorize foods as low, medium, or high GI in most circumstances. We have also found that many people who substitute low for high GI foods in their everyday meals and snacks reduce the overall GI of their diet, gain better blood glucose control, and lose weight.

You don't need to be pedantic about GI values

Whether a food's GI is 59 or 61 isn't biologically relevant. Normal day-to-day variation in the human body could obscure the difference in these values. Generally, a variation of more than 5 could be considered different.

This for that—substituting high GI with low GI foods

Simply substituting high GI foods with low GI alternatives will give your overall diet a lower GI and deliver the benefits of low GI eating. Here's how you can put slow carbs to work in your day by cutting back consumption of high GI foods and replacing them with alternatives that are just as tasty.

If you are currently eating this (high GI) food	Choose this (low GI) alternative instead
Cookies	A slice of whole-grain bread or toast with jam or fruit spread
Breads such as soft white or whole wheat; smooth textured breads, rolls, scones	Dense breads with whole grains, whole grain and stoneground flour, and sourdough
Breakfast cereals—most commercial, processed cereals including corn flakes, Rice Krispies, shredded wheat	Traditional rolled oats, muesli, and the commercial low GI brands listed in the tables. Look for the low GI symbol
Cakes and pastries	Raisin toast, fruit bread, and fruit buns are healthier baked options; yogurts and low fat pudding also make great snacks or desserts
Chips and other packaged snacks such as cheese curls, pretzels, potato sticks	Fresh fruits, dried apple, apricots, or dried fruit and nut mix
Crackers	Crisp vegetable strips such as carrot, pepper, or celery
Doughnuts and croissants	Skim milk cappuccino or smoothie

If you are currently eating this (high GI) food	Choose this (low GI) alternative instead
French fries	Leave them out! Have salad or extra vegetables instead. Corn on the cob or coleslaw are better takeout options
Candy	Chocolate is lower GI but high in fat. Healthier options are raisins, dried apricots, and other dried fruits
Muesli bars	Try a nut bar or dried fruit and nut mix. Look for the low GI symbol
Potatoes	Prepare smaller amounts of potato and add some sweet potato or sweet corn. Canned new potatoes are an easy and lower GI option. You can also try yam, taro, or just replace with other low GI or no-GI vegetables
Rice, especially large servings of it in dishes such as risotto, and fried rice	Try Basmati Converted Long Grain Rice, SunRice Low GI (white or brown), pearled barley, cracked wheat (bulgur), quinoa, pasta, or noodles. Look for the Low GI symbol
Soda and fruit juice drinks, like Kool-Aid and Hawaiian Punch	Use a diet variety if you drink these often. Fruit juice has a lower GI (but it is not a lower calorie option). Water or milk is best
Sugar	Moderate the quantity. Consider 100% pure wildflower honey, apple juice, and fructose as alternatives

Your GI Q&A

Does low carb automatically mean low GI?

Not at all. Low carb is *just about quantity*; it simply means that a food or meal does not contain much carbohydrate at all. It says nothing about the quality of the carbs in the food or meal on your plate. You could be eating a low carb meal, but the carbs have a medium or high GI. Low GI, on the other hand, is *all about quality*. Whether you are a moderate or high carb eater, low GI carbs (whole grain breads, legumes/beans, many fruits and vegetables) will have significant health benefits—promoting weight control, reducing your blood glucose and insulin levels throughout the day, and increasing your sense of feeling full and satisfied after eating. We suggest that you make the most of quality carbs and reap the add-on health benefits such as:

❏ Vitamin E from whole grain cereals

❏ Vitamin C, beta-carotene, and potassium from fruits and vegetables

❏ Vitamin B6 from bananas and whole grain cereals

❏ Pantothenic acid, zinc, iron, and magnesium from whole grains and legumes

❏ Antioxidants and phytochemicals from all plant foods

❏ Fiber, which comes from all of the above and doesn't come from any animal food

Why do many high-fiber foods have a high GI value?
Dietary fiber is not one chemical constituent like fat and protein. It is composed of many different sorts of molecules and can be divided into soluble and insoluble types. Soluble fiber is often viscous (thick and jelly-like) in solution and remains viscous even in the small intestine. For this reason it makes it harder for enzymes to move around and digest the food. Foods with more-soluble fiber, like apples, oats, and beans, therefore have low GI values.

Insoluble fiber, on the other hand, is not viscous and doesn't slow digestion unless it's acting like a fence to inhibit access by enzymes (e.g., the bran around intact kernels). When insoluble fiber is finely milled, the enzymes have free reign, allowing rapid digestion. Whole wheat bread and white bread have similar GI values. Brown pasta and brown rice have similar values to their white counterparts.

Should I avoid all high GI foods?
There is no need to eat only low GI foods. While you will benefit from eating low GI foods at each meal, this doesn't have to be to the exclusion of all others. When eaten with protein foods or low GI foods, the overall GI value of the meal will be about medium.

What GI number should a person aim for when trying to diet?

The simple answer is there's no formula. You don't need to add up the GI each day. In fact there's no counting at all as there is with calories. The basic technique for eating the low GI way is simply switching the high GI carbs in your diet with low GI foods. So, what you need to aim for is identifying the high GI carbs in your current diet and swapping them for some quality low GI carbs. When you're looking at GI values, it's best to compare like with like, one bread with another, for example, rather than "bread" with "fruit." This way you'll be comparing foods of similar nutritional value which will help you to make an appropriate swap from the high GI to the low GI version. Try keeping these simple guidelines in mind:

Every day you need to:

❏ Eat at least three meals—don't skip meals. Eat snacks, too, if you are hungry.

❏ Eat fruit at least twice—fresh, cooked, dried, juiced—aiming for at least 1½ cups per day.

❏ Eat vegetables at least twice—cooked, raw, salads, soups, juices, and snacks—aiming for at least 2½ cups per day.

❏ Eat a grain food at least once—bread, breakfast cereal, pasta, rice, noodles, and other grains such as barley, rye, oats, quinoa—in a whole grain or low GI form.

❏ Accumulate 60 minutes of physical activity (including incidental activity and planned exercise).

Every week you need to:

❏ Eat beans, peas, and/or lentils—at least twice (more often if you don't eat meat). This includes baked beans, chickpeas, red kidney beans, butter beans, split peas, and foods made from them such as hummus and dhal.

❏ Eat fish and seafood at least once, preferably three times, each week—fresh, smoked, frozen, or canned.

❏ Eat nuts regularly—just a tiny handful.

3 steps to a balanced low GI meal

1 is for carb
It's an essential, although sometimes maligned, part of a balanced meal. What do you feel like? A grain like rice, barley, or cracked wheat? Pasta, noodles, or bean vermicelli? Or perhaps a high carb vegetable like corn, sweet potato, or legumes? Include at least one low GI carb per meal.

2 is for protein
Include some protein at each meal. It lowers the glycemic load by replacing *some* of the carbohydrate—not all! It also helps satisfy the appetite.

3 is for fruit and vegetables
This is the part we often go without. If anything it should have the highest priority in a meal, but a meal based solely on fruit and low carb vegetables won't be sustaining for long. A plain salad sandwich is a recipe for hunger.

What's a serving?

Indulgences
2 tablespoons cream, sour cream
1 oz chocolate
1 small slice (about 1½ oz) cake
1 small bag (1 oz) potato chips
2 standard alcoholic drinks (a 5-oz glass of wine, 1½ oz of distilled spirits, or a 12-oz beer)

Fish, seafood, lean meats, poultry, eggs & alternatives
3 oz (cooked) boneless meat, fish, or chicken
3 oz canned fish
2 eggs
1½ oz reduced-fat cheese or 1 oz full-fat cheese
3½ oz tofu

Legumes
½ cup cooked lentils, chickpeas, beans

Low fat dairy or alternative
1 cup milk or soy milk
1 cup yogurt

Nuts & oils
2 teaspoons olive or canola oil
1 tablespoon oil-based vinaigrette
½ oz nuts
¼ cup avocado

Breads, cereals, rice, pasta, noodles, grains
1 slice bread
½ cup cooked rice, pasta, or noodles
½ cup cereal

Fruit & juices
1 medium piece of fruit
1 cup small fruit pieces
½ cup juice

Vegetables
½ cup cooked vegetables
1 cup raw or salad vegetables

Low GI
shopping

Planning to shop

The perfect place to get started on healthy low GI eating is the supermarket, whether you are pushing a cart up and down the aisles or shopping online. This is where we make those hurried or impulsive decisions that have a big impact.

Spend a little time each day, or weekly if it suits, planning what to eat when. It makes life simpler. Meal planning is just writing down what you intend to eat for the main meals of the week, then checking your fridge and pantry for ingredients available and noting what you need to purchase.

Our shopping list on pages 24 to 35 will help you stock the pantry and fridge with the staples you require to turn out a meal in minutes. To make your own shopping list, use the same headings. They will take you to the appropriate aisles of the supermarket or to the shops you usually favor. We've included convenience foods such as canned beans, bagged salads, bottled sauces and pastes, canned fruits, and chopped vegetables (fresh and frozen) in the list. There's no need to feel guilty about using these items. Although some convenience items such as frozen vegetables or canned beans may be a little more expensive, the time savings and health benefits can outweigh the costs.

Making sense of food labeling

Often we're asked questions like: "What should I look for on the label?" and "Can I believe what it says?" There's lots of information on food labels these days, but unfortunately, very few people know how to interpret it correctly. Often the claims on the front of the package don't mean quite what you think.

Here are some prime examples:

Natural—tends to make us feel good about the food but it has no formal definition (except in relation to meat).

Cholesterol free—doesn't necessarily mean heart-healthy. It could still be loaded with excess amounts of fat, sugar, and salt.

Whole grain—check the ingredient list to look for 100% whole grain

Now with less fat—take care, if fat has been removed, what has been added? Sometimes good fats are replaced by refined starches and sugars.

Understanding the Nutrition Facts Panel

To get the hard facts on the nutritional value of a food, take a closer look at the Nutrition Facts Panel. This is where you'll find the details regarding the fat, calories, carbohydrate, fiber, and sodium content of the food.

These are the key points to look for:

Serving size—This is the amount of food on which the nutrition values are based, so compare this to the amount you actually eat.

Calories—Check total calories and aim for less if you want to manage your weight.

Saturated fats, trans fat, cholesterol, and sodium—Your aim ought to be to limit these. Indeed, trans fat should be zero. Check the ingredient list and avoid foods made with partially hydrogenated oils. Use the %DV (daily value) as a framework. A quick guide: a %DV of 5% or less is low and 20% or more is high.

Total carbohydrate—This is the starch + sugars + fiber. You can estimate usable carbohydrate by subtracting fiber from the total carbohydrate content. This is used to calculate the glycemic load. (See pages 50–51 for more information about GL.)

Total sugar/added sugar—Sugars in food may be naturally occurring as in fruit and vegetables or "added" as in soda. An apple contains as much as 12g per 100 g—the same as soda. Added (or free) sugars are those added by the manufacturer, including cane sugar and HFCS. The role of added sugars is controversial, but most authorities say that 7–9 teaspoons a day (30–50 grams) will *not* cause harm.

Fiber—This is the nondigestible part of carbohydrate that is so important to the health of our gut. It's something most of us don't get enough of. Remember 5% DV is low fiber, 20% DV or more is high.

Sodium—Our bodies need some salt, but most people consume far more than they need. Over 75% of the sodium we eat comes from packaged foods, so it is important to check the figures. A low-sodium food would have 140mg or less per serving.

YOUR SHOPPING LIST

The bakery

❑ Fruit bread
❑ Low GI bread
    Whole grain
    Sourdough
    Soy and Flaxseed
❑ English muffins
❑ Pita bread

The refrigerator case

❑ Cheese
    Cottage cheese / ricotta, reduced fat
    Grated cheese, reduced fat
    Parmesan cheese
    Sliced cheese, reduced fat
❑ Dairy desserts
    Custard, low fat
    Mousse, low fat
❑ Dips
    Hummus
❑ Fruit juice
    Apple juice
    Cranberry juice

 Look out for this shopping cart icon on the following pages for ways to cut your food budget and increase your healthy eating habits.

Grapefruit juice
Orange juice

 Look for fruit juices that are "100% pure" and "unsweetened." And remember not to overdo it— one serving is ½ cup.

❑ Margarine, canola-based
❑ Milk
    Low fat
    Low fat, flavored
    Skim
❑ Noodles, fresh

 Many Asian noodles, such as "wet" egg noodles, udon, and rice vermicelli, have low to intermediate GI values because of their processing, whether they are made from wheat or rice flour.

❑ Pasta, fresh
    Ravioli
    Tortellini
❑ Soy products
    Soy milk, low fat, calcium-enriched
    Soy yogurt
    Soy frozen dessert
❑ Sushi
❑ Tofu
❑ Yogurt

 Low fat natural yogurt provides the most calcium for the fewest calories. Have vanilla or fruit

versions as a dessert, or use natural yogurt as a
condiment in savory dishes.

Drinkable yogurt, low fat
Fruit or vanilla flavored, low fat
Plain/natural, low fat

The freezer

❑ Frozen berries

Berries can make any dessert special. Using
frozen ones means you don't have to wait until
berry season.

Blueberries
Raspberries
Strawberries

❑ Frozen fruit desserts or gelato
❑ Frozen vegetables

Frozen vegetables are handy to add to a
quick meal.

Beans
Broccoli
Cauliflower
Corn
Mixed vegetables
Peas
Spinach
Stir-fry mix

❏ Frozen yogurt

Frozen yogurt is a fantastic substitute for ice cream. Some products even have a similar creamy texture, but with much less fat.

❏ Ice cream
Vanilla or flavored, reduced or low fat

Fresh fruit and vegetables

❏ Basics
Carrots
Chili peppers
Corn on the cob
Garlic
Ginger
Lemons or limes
Onions
Sweet potato
Taro
Yam

❏ Fruit, depending on season
Apples
Apricots
Grapefruit
Grapes
Mango
Oranges
Peaches

Pears

Strawberries

❏ Herbs, fresh, depending on season

Fresh herbs are available in most supermarkets
and there really is no substitute for the flavor they
impart.

Basil

Chives

Cilantro

Mint

Parsley

❏ Leafy green and other seasonal vegetables

Pile your plate high with leafy greens and eat your
way to long-term health.

Asian greens, such as bok choy

Asparagus

Beans

Broccoli

Brussels sprouts

Cabbage

Cauliflower

Eggplant

Fennel

Kale

Leeks

Mushrooms

Snow peas

Spinach
Squash
Zucchini
❑ Salad vegetables, depending on season
Arugula
Avocado
Bagged mixed salad greens
Celery
Cucumber
Lettuce
Pepper
Spring onions
Sprouts, such as mung bean, snow pea, alfalfa
Tomato

General groceries

❑ Beverages
Coffee
Flavored milk powders, such as Nesquik®
Tea
❑ Breakfast cereals
Low GI packaged breakfast cereal
Natural muesli
Rolled oats, traditional

 Besides their use in oatmeal, oats can be added to cakes, cookies, breads, and desserts.

❏ Canned foods
 Baked beans
 Beans, such as cannellini, butter, black, lima,
  kidney, chickpeas, etc.
 Corn kernels
 Four bean mix
 Lentils
 Mexi-beans
 Salmon, in water
 Sardines
 Skim milk, evaporated

 **Canned evaporated skim milk makes an
 excellent substitute for cream in pasta sauces.**

 Tomatoes, whole, crushed

 **Tomatoes can be used freely because they are
 rich in antioxidants, as well as having a low GI.**

 Tomato paste
 Tomato soup
 Tuna, in spring water or oil

❏ Canned fruit

 **Have a variety of canned fruit on hand—choose
 the brands labeled with "no added sugar" fruit
 juice syrup.**

 Mixed fruit salad

Peaches

Pears

❑ Cereals and whole grains

Barley, pearl

One of the oldest cultivated cereals, barley is very nutritious and high in fiber. Look for products such as pearl barley to use in soups, stews, and pilafs.

Bulgur/cracked wheat

Use bulgur to make tabbouleh, or add to vegetable burgers, stuffings, soups, and stews.

Couscous

Couscous can be ready in minutes; serve with casseroles and braised dishes.

Noodles

Pasta

Pasta is a great source of carbohydrates and B vitamins.

Rice, such as Basmati, SunRice Low GI (white or brown)

Quinoa

Quinoa cooks in about 10–15 minutes and has a slightly chewy texture. It can be used as a substitute for rice, couscous, or bulgur wheat. It is very important to rinse the grains thoroughly before cooking.

❏ Condiments

Asian sauces

Hoisin, oyster, soy, and fish sauces are a good range of Asian sauces.

Black pepper
Chili pepper, minced
Curry paste
Dried herbs
Garlic, minced
Ginger, minced
Horseradish cream
Mustard
Pasta sauce
Sea salt
Soy sauce
Spices
Tomato sauce

❏ Dried fruit and nuts
   Apple rings
   Apricots
   Natural almonds, walnuts, cashews, unsalted
   Prunes
   Raisins
❏ Dried legumes
   Beans

   Keep a variety of beans in the cupboard including cannellini, black, lima, kidney, soy, pinto.

   Chickpeas
   Lentils
   Split peas
❏ Deli items or prepacked jars
   Anchovies
   Capers
   Eggplant
   Olives
   Peppers
   Sundried tomatoes
❏ Eggs

   Buy omega-3-enriched eggs. They are a good way of boosting your omega-3 intake, particularly if you don't eat fish.

❑ Oils and vinegars

    Canola is good for high temperature frying

    Specialty oils like walnut, macadamia, and sesame are
        great for added flavor

    Olive oil, preferably extra virgin, especially for salad
        dressing and marinades

 **Try olive oil for general use; use extra-virgin
olive oil for salad dressings, marinades, and
dishes that benefit from its flavor.**

    Vinegar, balsamic and white wine

❑ Spreads

    Honey

 **Avoid the honey blends, and use 100% "pure
floral" honeys, which have a much lower GI.**

    Jam

 **A dollop of good-quality jam on toast contains
fewer calories than butter or margarine.**

    Peanut butter, natural

Butcher/meat department

❑ Bacon

 **Bacon is a valuable ingredient in many dishes
because of the flavor it offers. You can make a
little bacon go a long way by trimming off all fat
and chopping it finely. Lean ham is often a more
economical and leaner way to go.**

- ❏ Beef, lean
- ❏ Chicken
    Skinless chicken breast or drumsticks
- ❏ Fish
    Any type of fresh fish
- ❏ Ground beef, lean
- ❏ Ham, lean
- ❏ Lamb fillets, lean
- ❏ Pork fillets, lean

Shopping & storage tips

Cheese

Any reduced fat cheese is great to keep handy in the fridge. A block of Parmesan is indispensable and will keep for up to a month. Reduced fat cottage and ricotta cheeses have a short life so are best bought as needed. They can be a good alternative to butter or margarine in a sandwich.

Vegetables and fruit

Vegetables are best fresh, so shop two or three times a week if you can and use them within a few days.

Ethylene gas produced by aging fruit and vegetables leads to their deterioration. You can minimize the effect of ethylene by storing vegetables in the fridge in long-life bags, which are available in the produce section of supermarkets, or you can use special cartridges (available in some supermarkets) designed to absorb ethylene. Fruits give off more ethylene than vegetables, but vegetables are more sensitive to its effects, so if you have two crispers, keep fruit in one and vegetables in the other.

Legumes and beans

Whether you buy them dried or opt for canned convenience, you are choosing one of nature's lowest GI foods. They are high in fiber and packed with nutrients, providing protein, carbohydrate, B vitamins, folate, and minerals. When you add legumes to meals and snacks, you reduce the overall GI of your diet because your body digests them slowly. This is primarily because their starch breaks down relatively slowly (or incompletely) during cooking and they contain tannins and enzyme inhibitors that also slow digestion.

Although they have an excellent shelf life, old beans take longer to cook than young, which is why it's a good idea to buy them from shops where you know turnover is brisk. Once home, store them in airtight containers in a cool, dry place—they will keep their color better.

Preparing dried legumes

1. **Wash** Wash thoroughly in a colander or sieve first, keeping an eye out for any small stones or "foreign" material (especially with lentils).
2. **Soak** Soaking plumps the beans, makes them softer and tastier, and reduces cooking times a little. Place them in a saucepan, cover with about three times their volume of cold water and soak overnight or for at least four hours. As a rule of thumb, the larger the seed, the longer the soaking time required. There's no need to soak lentils or split peas.
3. **Cook** Drain, rinse thoroughly, then add fresh water—two to three times the volume of the legumes. Bring to a boil then reduce the heat

and simmer until tender. Generally, you will need to simmer lentils and peas for 45–60 minutes and beans and chickpeas for 1–2 hours, but check the recipe instructions. A couple of points to keep in mind:

❏ Adding salt to the water during cooking will slow down water absorption and the legumes will take longer to cook.

❏ Make sure that legumes are tender before you add acidic flavorings such as lemon juice or tomatoes. Once they are in an acid medium, they won't get any softer no matter how long you cook them.

Time-saving tips

❏ If you don't have time to soak legumes overnight, add three times the volume of water to rinsed beans, bring to a boil for a few minutes, and then remove from the heat and soak for an hour. Drain, rinse, and add fresh water; then cook as usual.

❏ Cooked legumes freeze well. Prepare a large quantity of beans or chickpeas and freeze in small batches to use as required.

❏ Store soaked or cooked beans in an airtight container in the fridge. They will keep for several days.

Noodles

You can buy noodles fresh, dried, or boiled (wet). Fresh and boiled noodles will be in the refrigerated section in your supermarket or Asian grocery store. Use them as soon as possible after purchase or store in the refrigerator for a day or two. Dried noodles are handy to have in the pantry for quick and easy meals in minutes. They will keep for several months, provided you haven't opened the package. Egg noodles are made from wheat flour and eggs. They are readily available dried, and you can find fresh egg noodles in the refrigerator section of the supermarket or Asian grocery store. "Wet" egg noodles will be in the refrigerated section too. Instant noodles are usually precooked and dehydrated egg noodles. Check the label as they are sometimes fried.

Spices

Most spices, including ground cumin, turmeric, cinnamon, paprika, and nutmeg, should be bought in small quantities because they lose pungency with age and incorrect storage. Keep them in dark, airtight containers.

Your shopping Q&A

How can I feed a big family with cost-effective, no-hassle low GI foods?

Feeding a big family on a budget can be hard. But low GI eating often means making a move back to the inexpensive, filling, and healthy staple foods that our parents and grandparents enjoyed. This includes traditional oats for oatmeal, legumes such as beans, chickpeas, and lentils (available in cans), cereal grains like barley, and of course plenty of fresh vegetables and fruit, which naturally have a low GI. Some of these foods may take a little more time to prepare than high GI processed, packaged, and pricey "convenience" foods piled high on supermarket shelves, but the savings will be considerable and the health benefits immeasurable. For a list of the top 100 low GI foods, check out *The New Glucose Revolution Low GI Eating Made Easy*. This book also includes plenty of ideas for using these foods in everyday meals.

I have recently been diagnosed with celiac disease or gluten intolerance. Any suggestions for foods that are both low GI and gluten-free?

This is not as hard as you may think. If you like Asian food—Indian dhals, stir-fries with rice, sushi, noodles—you're in luck, because they are all low GI. Choose vermicelli noodles prepared from rice or mung beans and low GI rices such as basmati or SunRice Low GI rice. Use sweet potato or Carisma potatoes, if available, instead of white potato. Use all manner of vegetables without any regard for their GI. Choose fruits and dairy for their low GI. If you can tolerate dairy products, then take advantage of them for their universal low GI. If lactose intolerance is a problem, reach for live cultured yogurts and lactose-hydrolyzed milks. Even ice cream can be enjoyed if you ingest a few drops of lactase enzyme (Lactaid) first.

I love to bake. If I make my own bread (or dumplings, pancakes, muffins, etc.), which flours, if any, are low GI?

There are no GI ratings for refined flour, whether it's made from wheat, soy, or other grains. This is because the GI rating of a food must be tested physiologically, that is, in real people. So far we haven't had volunteers willing to tuck into about 2 oz (or ½ cup) of raw flour! What we do know, however, is that bakery products such as scones, cakes, biscuits, doughnuts, and pastries made from refined flour, whether it's white or whole wheat, are quickly digested and absorbed.

What should you do with your own baking? Try to increase the soluble fiber content by partially substituting flour with oat bran, rice bran, or rolled oats and increase the bulkiness of the product with dried fruit, nuts, muesli, All-Bran, or unprocessed bran. Don't think of it as a challenge. It's an opportunity for some creative cooking. See some of our recipes in *The Low GI Diet Cookbook, The New Glucose Revolution Low GI Vegetarian Cookbook,* and *The New Glucose Revolution Low GI Family Cookbook.*

Low GI Breads and Breakfast Cereals

Did you know that the type of bread and cereal you eat affects the overall GI of your diet the most? Why? Well, cereal grains such as rice, wheat, oats, barley, and rye and products made from them such as bread and breakfast cereals are the most concentrated sources of carbohydrate in our diet.

A simple swap is all it takes to reduce the GI of your diet. To get started, replace some of those high GI breads and breakfast cereals with low GI carbs that will trickle fuel into your engine. Here's a list of some of the low GI breads and breakfast cereals you will find in your local supermarket or shopping center.

Breads	GI
3 grain bread, sprouted grains	55
100% whole grain bread	51
COBS High Fiber, Low GI Bread	46
corn tortilla	52
flaxseed and soy bread	55
President's Choice Blue Menu Whole Grain English Muffin	51
pumpernickel bread	50
sourdough rye bread	48
sourdough wheat bread	54
spelt multigrain bread	54
Country Life, Low GI Gluten-Free Bread	40

Breakfast cereals and bars	GI
Cereals	
All-Bran, Kellogg's, original	50
Frosted Flakes, Kellogg's	55
Muesli, natural	40
Oatmeal, from steel-cut oats, made with water	52
Oatmeal, multigrain, dry packet	55
President's Choice Blue Menu Fiberfirst Multi-bran Cereal	55
President's Choice Blue Menu Omega-3 granola cereal	43
Bars	
Balance Bar Gold Caramel Nut Blast	17
Balance Bar Original Peanut Butter	25
Luna Cookie Dough Bar	18
Nutrisystem Apple Granola Bar	52
SoLo GI Energy Bar Mint Mania	23
SoLo GI Energy Bar Peanut Power	27
Biscuits	
belVita, Breakfast Biscuits, Crunchy Oats	54
belVita, Breakfast Biscuits, Fruit & Fiber	47
belVita, Breakfast Biscuits, Milk & Cereal	45

How do you know if it's truly low GI?

In Australia, the GI symbol makes healthy shopping easier. This symbol means that the food has been assessed by the experts. It's your guarantee that the GI value stated near the nutrition information table is reliable.

Foods that carry the certified GI symbol have also been judged against a range of nutrient criteria so you can be sure that the food is a healthy nutritional choice for its food group.

Our American cousins should demand a similar program in their country.

Why put the GI symbol on food labels?
Before 2001, people had to rely on published lists of the glycemic index of foods to help them decide which carbohydrate foods to eat. The GI symbol helps

identify healthy foods that have a GI value, making it much easier for you to choose foods on the basis of their GI.

Which foods carry the GI symbol?
Low GI foods carry the symbol, provided they meet the nutrient criteria. The symbol identifies foods that have had their GI tested properly, and that are a healthy choice for their food category. The GI ranking (low) is stated within the symbol, and the GI value is specified near the nutrition information panel. To carry the GI symbol, the food has to be independently tested following a standardized international method.

Is the GI symbol an indication that foods are healthy?
Foods with the Glycemic Index symbol are healthy in other respects. To earn the certification, foods must be a good source of carbohydrate and meet a host of other nutrient criteria including calories, total and saturated fat, sodium (salt), and, when appropriate, dietary fiber and calcium.

Are foods with the GI symbol good for people with diabetes?
If you have diabetes, you need to consider the quantity of carbohydrate in your serving of food, as well as the GI. Calculating the glycemic load (GL) (grams of carbohydrate $\times$ GI $\div 100$) is one way of combining both factors. (See pages 50–51 for more information on the GL.)

How can we be sure the information is accurate?

Foods in the program are required to undergo re-testing for their GI if there is any change in product formulation. All product labels and advertising that use the symbol or mention the program are preapproved by the Glycemic Index Foundation. The Foundation is not responsible, though, for the accuracy and legality of labels and marketing claims of the foods in the program.

Who is Glycemic Index Limited?

The Glycemic Index Foundation is a not-for-profit health promotion charity supported by the University of Sydney, Diabetes Australia, and the Juvenile Diabetes Research Foundation. It represents Australia's peak body of glycemic index research and education. Manufacturers pay the Glycemic Index Foundation a license fee to use the certified GI symbol on their products, and the income is channeled back into education and research.

Why don't all low GI foods have the symbol?

A food may make a low GI claim on its label, yet not carry the symbol. It may have been tested correctly (check the tables or the online database at www.glycemicindex.com, or contact the food manufacturer to double-check), but the manufacturer may choose not to participate in the GI Symbol Program. Also, the food might not meet the other nutritional guidelines as it may be high in calories, total or saturated fat, or sodium, or low in fiber or calcium—check the Nutrition Facts panel.

What about other labels that claim a food is low GI? Can I trust them?

Claims about the GI of foods are currently not regulated. Manufacturers are free to make claims provided they are not false or misleading. They should print the GI value of the food on the food label to help you to verify the claim. A food with a low GI should have a value less than or equal to 55. There are a number of brands that make low GI claims but do not provide a GI value or definition of what low GI means on the label. Unfortunately, you have no way of verifying whether the claim is legitimate. Without verification, it's probably sensible not to trust the claim because you have no idea whether the food was tested following the standardized procedure by an accredited lab.

Sometimes a GI value may be too low to be true. If a manufacturer is promoting a carb-rich processed food with an ultra low GI and does not carry the certified GI symbol, be wary before you buy. Processed foods such as breakfast cereals and breads and bakery products are very unlikely to have a very low GI. In fact, if the GI is less than, say, 50, we suggest that you ask the manufacturer for the name of the lab that tested it and the method that was used.

You may also see products claiming to be "low glycemic" or "diabetic friendly," leaving it open as to whether it's low GI, low GL, or low glycemic response. Be cautious with these claims as the product could actually be low carb (check the nutrition label). Manufacturers making these claims may not be intending to mislead the consumer;

they simply may not understand the difference. It's useful to write and ask what they mean and where the food was tested. There are a number of foods that use low GI logos that are similar to the Glycemic Index Tested logo. Some of these cases have been pursued through legal channels.

❏ Consumers in the USA and Canada can contact the Food and Drug Administration's Office of Compliance at the Center for Food Safety and Applied Nutrition (for the USA) and the Canadian Food Inspection Agency (for Canada).

For more information about the Glycemic Index Symbol Program and the latest list of approved products, go to www.gisymbol.com.au.

How we determine a food's GI value

The GI is a scale from 0 to 100 that captures how the carbohydrates in foods affect blood glucose levels ("glycemia"). It's based on testing real foods in real people. To make an absolutely fair comparison, all foods are tested following an internationally standardized method. The higher the GI, the higher the blood glucose levels after consumption of a standard amount. The GI rating of a food must be tested physiologically, and only a few centers around the world currently provide a legitimate testing service.

Testing the GI of a food requires a group of ten subjects and knowledge of the food's carbohydrate content. After an overnight fast, each subject consumes a portion of the test food containing a specified amount of carbohydrate (usually 50 grams, but sometimes 25 or even 15 grams). Finger-prick blood samples are taken at 15- to 30-minute intervals over the next two hours. During this time, blood glucose levels rise and fall back to baseline levels. The full extent of glycemia (rise in blood glucose) is assessed by measuring the area under the curve using a computer algorithm.

There will be some variation between subjects, but if we were to test them again and again, all subjects would tend to move toward the average of the whole group.

What is the glycemic load?

Your blood glucose rises and falls when you eat a food or meal containing carbohydrate. How high it rises and how long it remains high depends on the quality of the carbohydrate (its glycemic index value, or GI) as well as the quantity of carbohydrate in your meal. Researchers at Harvard University came up with a term that combines these two factors—glycemic load (GL).

Some people think that GL should be used instead of GI when comparing foods because it reflects the glycemic impact of both the quantity and quality of carbohydrate in a food. But more often than not, it's low GI (not low GL) that predicts good health outcomes, the reason being that following the low glycemic load (GL) route can lead you straight to a low carb diet: for example, fatty meats and butter have a low GL. But if you eat plenty of low GI foods, you'll find that you are automatically reducing the GL of your diet and, at the same time, you'll feel fuller for longer.

We also emphasize that there's no need to get overly technical about this. Think of the GI as a tool allowing you to choose one food over another in the same food group—the best bread to choose, the best cereal to choose, etc.—and don't get bogged down with figures. A low GI diet is about eating a wide variety of healthy foods that fuel our bodies best—on the whole these are the less processed and more wholesome foods that will provide carbs in a slow release form.

The glycemic load is calculated simply by multiplying the GI value of a food by the amount of carbohydrate per serving and dividing by 100.

Here's how:

$$\text{Glycemic load} = (GI \times \text{carbohydrate per serving}) \div 100$$

Let's say you wanted to have an apple for a snack. Apples have a GI of 38, and one medium apple contains 15 grams of carbohydrate. So, the glycemic load of your apple snack is $(38 \times 15) \div 100 = 6$.

If you were very hungry and ate two apples, you would be eating 30 grams of carbs and the GL of your snack would be 12. The GI doesn't change, but you are eating more carbs because you are eating two apples.

Top 10 carbs for kids

1 Oatmeal: A sustaining start to the day—add in raisins or banana slices.

2 Yogurt: Sweetened or not, it's a great source of calcium and protein.

3 Whole grain toast: Spread with peanut butter and jelly, it makes a far healthier snack than cookies.

4 Fruit bread: A slice of dense fruit toast spread with ricotta cheese

5 Apple: Ideal for the lunch box or sliced as a snack.

6 Canned fruits: Portable snack packs are perfect when out and about.

7 Dried fruits: Colorful and sweet, with added nuts and seeds if you like.

8 Corn: Perfect on the cob and a great addition to mixed veggies.

9 Popcorn: Best made yourself where you can control any added fats and salt.

10 Sweet potato: Steamed, mashed, or roasted, a great alternative to the traditional spud.

Eating
out

Eating out the low GI way

Whether you think it is compatible with healthy eating or not, statistics tell us that at some point you are going to be eating out or buying take-out food. Eating out can really test your resolve as far as healthy eating goes. Like any food choice, however, the more often we eat out, the more important it is that we choose healthy options. If you only eat out once a month, you needn't be too fussy, but if it's three to four times a week, good choices are critical.

Finding the low GI choice on the menu

Indian food

The traditional accompaniment for Indian dishes is steamed basmati rice, which is a classic low GI choice. Lentil dhal offers another lower GI accompaniment, but make sure they don't add the oil topping (tadka).

Unleavened breads such as chapati or roti may have a lower GI than normal bread, but they will boost the carbohydrate content of the meal and increase the GL.

Our suggestions:

❏ Tikka (dry roasted) or tandoori (marinated in spices and yogurt) chicken

❏ Basmati rice

❏ Cucumber raita

❏ Spicy spinach (saag)

Japanese food

Sushi has a low GI, and any refrigerated rice has a lower GI than when it is freshly cooked. The vinegar used in preparation of sushi helps keep the GI low (acidity helps slow stomach emptying), and so do the viscous fibers in the seaweed. Typical ingredients and flavors to enjoy are shoyu (Japanese soy sauce), mirin (rice wine), wasabi (a strong horseradish), miso (soybean paste), pickled ginger (oshinko), sesame seeds, and sesame oil. Go easy on deep-fried dishes such as tempura.

Japanese restaurants are great places to stock up on omega-3 fats, as dishes such as sushi and sashimi made with salmon and tuna contain high amounts of beneficial polyunsaturated fatty acids.

Our suggestions:

❑ Miso soup

❑ Edamame beans

❑ Sushi

❑ Teppanyaki (steak, seafood, and vegetables)

❑ Yakitori (skewered chicken and onions in teriyaki sauce)

❑ Sashimi (thinly sliced raw fish or beef)

❑ Shabu-shabu (thin slices of beef quickly cooked with mushrooms, cabbage, and other vegetables)

❑ Side orders such as seaweed salad, wasabi, soy sauce, and pickled ginger

Thai food

Thai food is generally sweet and spicy and contains aromatic ingredients such as basil, lemongrass, and galangal. Spicy Thai salads, which usually contain seafood, chicken, or meat, are a delicious light meal. For starters, avoid the deep-fried items such as spring rolls.

One downside to Thai cuisine is the coconut milk, which really raises the saturated fat content of Thai curry. So don't feel you have to consume all of the sauce or soup. The traditional accompaniment to Thai food is plain, steamed Jasmine rice, but this is very high GI so you are better off if you can reduce the quantity. Noodles are always on the menu as well, but avoid fried versions. Boiled rice noodles may be an option. Limit yourself to a small helping, or if you are having takeout, you could cook up some long grain rice at home as an accompaniment.

Our suggestions:

❑ Tom yum—hot and sour soup

❑ Thai beef or chicken salad

❑ Wok-tossed meats or seafood

❑ Stir-fried mixed vegetables

❑ Small serving of steamed noodles or rice

❑ Fresh spring rolls (not fried)

Italian food

The big plus with Italian restaurants is the supply of low GI pasta with an array of sauces. Good choices are arrabiata, puttanesca, marinara sauces (without cream). Despite what you may think, most Italians don't sit down to huge bowls of pasta, so don't be afraid to leave some on your plate (or order an appetizer size)—the GI may be low but a large serving of pasta will have a high GL. Other good choices include minestrone and vegetable dishes, lean veal, and grilled seafood. Steer clear of crumbed and deep-fried seafood.

Our suggestions:

❏ Minestrone

❏ Veal scallops in tomato-based sauce

❏ Prosciutto (paper-thin slices of smoky ham) wrapped around melon

❏ Barbecued or grilled seafood such as calamari or octopus

❏ Roasted or grilled fillet of beef, lamb loin, or poultry

❏ Green garden salad with olive oil and balsamic vinegar

❏ Sorbet, gelato, or simply a fresh fruit platter

❏ Appetizer-size pasta with seafood and tomato or stock-based sauce

Greek and Middle Eastern food

In Mediterranean cuisine, olive oil, lemon, garlic, onions, and other vegetables abound. Many dishes are char-grilled and specialities such as barbecued octopus or grilled sardines are excellent choices. You will find regular bread replaced with flat bread or Turkish bread, while potatoes are replaced with healthier options such as bulgur (in tabbouleh) and couscous. Among the small appetizing mezze dishes, you could pick and choose what you like. Many of the choices are healthy, such as hummus, baba ghanoush, olives, tzatziki, and grape leaves.

Our suggestions:

❑ Mezze platter with Lebanese bread

❑ Souvlaki (grilled skewers of meat with vegetables)

❑ Kofta (balls of minced lamb with bulgur wheat)

❑ Greek salad of fresh lettuce, tomato, olives, feta, and peppers, with balsamic dressing or oil and lemon

❑ Fresh fruit platter

❑ Falafel with tabbouleh and hummus with a flat bread

Tips for those who routinely eat at restaurants

1 *Walk* to the restaurant if possible.
2 Order water as soon as you arrive.
3 Send the bread basket away (unless it's *exceptional*).
4 Order green salad, raw oysters, or soup for an appetizer.
5 Order an appetizer for your main course (or specify appetizer size).
6 Alternatively, eat *only half* of everything on your plate.
7 Tell the waiter to hold the French fries.
8 Share dessert with a dining companion.
9 Drink no more than one or two glasses of alcohol.
10 Walk back to the office or climb the stairs instead of taking the elevator or escalator.

Fast-food outlets

Burgers and French fries are a bad idea—quickly eaten, high in saturated fat, and rapidly absorbed high GI carbs that fill you with calories that don't last long. Some fast-food chains are introducing healthier choices, but read the fine print. Look out for lean protein, low GI carbs, good fats, and lots of vegetables.

Our suggestions:

❑ Marinated and barbecued chicken, rather than fried

❑ Salads such as coleslaw or garden salad; eat the salad first

❑ Corn on the cob as a healthy side order

❑ Individual menu items rather than meal deals—never upsize

❑ Mexican dishes based on beans and rice—but go easy on the cheese

Lunch bars

Steer clear of places displaying lots of deep-fried fare and head toward fresh food bars offering fruit and vegetables. Tubs of garden or Greek salad topped with fruit and yogurt make a healthy, low GI choice.

With sandwiches and melts, choose the fillings carefully. Including cheese can make the fat exceed 20 grams per sandwich (that's as much as French fries!). Make sure you include some vegetables or salad in or alongside the sandwich.

Our suggestions:

- ❏ Dense grain bread rather than white
- ❏ Salad fillings for sandwiches, or as a side order instead of fries
- ❏ Pasta dishes with both vegetables and meat
- ❏ Lebanese kebabs with tabbouleh and hummus
- ❏ Grilled fish rather than fried
- ❏ Vegetarian pizza
- ❏ Gourmet wraps

Cafés

Whether it's a quick snack or a main meal, catching up with a friend for coffee doesn't have to tip your diet off balance. Pass on breads, but if you really must, something like a dense Italian bread is better than a garlic or herb bread.

Whatever you order, specify: "no French fries—extra salad instead" so temptation does not confront you. If you want something sweet, try a skim iced cappuccino or a single little cookie or a small piece of sponge cake.

Our suggestions:

- ❏ Skim milk coffee rather than full cream milk
- ❏ Sourdough or whole-grain bread instead of white or whole wheat
- ❏ Bruschetta with tomatoes, onions, olive oil, and basil on a dense Italian bread rather than buttery herb or garlic bread

❑ Salad as a main or side order, with the dressing served separately so you control the amount

❑ Grilled steak or chicken breast rather than fried or battered

❑ Vegetable-topped pizza—such as pepper, onion, mushroom, artichoke, eggplant

❑ Lean meat pizza—such as ham, fresh seafood, or sliced chicken breast

❑ Pasta with sauces such as marinara; meat sauce; puttanesca; arrabiata (tomato with olives, roasted pepper, and chili); and piccolo (eggplant, roasted pepper, and artichoke)

❑ Seafood such as marinated calamari, grilled with chili and lemon, or steamed mussels with a tomato sauce

❑ Water or freshly squeezed fruit and vegetable juices rather than soft drinks

Asian meals

Asian meals, including Chinese, Thai, Indian, and Japanese, offer a great variety of foods, making it possible to select a healthy meal with some careful choices.

Keeping in line with the 1, 2, 3 steps to a balanced meal (see page 16), seek out a lower GI carb such as basmati rice, dhal, sushi, or noodles. Chinese and Thai rice will traditionally be jasmine, and, although high GI, a small serving of steamed rice is better for you than fried rice or noodles.

Next add some protein—marinated tofu (bean curd), stir-fried seafood, Tandoori chicken, fish tikka, or a braised dish with vegetables. Be cautious with pork and duck, for which fattier cuts are often used; and avoid Thai curries and dishes made with coconut milk because it's high in saturated fat.

And don't forget, the third dish to order is stir-fried vegetables!

Our suggestions:

❏ Steamed dumplings or fresh spring rolls rather than fried entrees

❏ Clear soups to fill you up rather than high fat coconut-based soups

❏ Noodles in soups rather than fried in dishes such as pad Thai

❏ Noodle and vegetable stir-fries—if you ask for extra vegetables you may find that the one dish feeds two

❏ Seafood braised in a sauce with vegetables

❏ Tofu, chicken, beef, lamb, or pork fillet braised with nuts, vegetables, black bean, or other sauces

❏ Salads such as Thai salads

❏ Smaller servings of rice

❏ Vegetable dishes such as stir-fried vegetables, vegetable curry, dhal, channa (a delicious chickpea curry), and side orders such as pickles, cucumber and yogurt, tomato and onion

❏ Japanese dishes such as sushi, teriyaki, sashimi, salmon steak or tuna, teppanyaki (which is grilled) in preference to tempura, which is deep-fried

Airlines and airports

Airports are notoriously bad places to eat. Fast-food chains, a limited range, premade sandwiches, sad-looking cakes, a lack of fresh fruit and vegetables, and it's all expensive!

In airline lounges you will do better, although, again, the range is limited. Fresh fruit is always on offer and usually some sort of vegetables, either as salad or soup. The bread is usually the super-high GI white French type and with crackers as the only other option, you would do better to rely on fruit, fruit juices, yogurt, or a skim milk coffee for your carbs.

In-flight, unless you have the privilege of a sky chef, meals are fairly standard fare, including a salad and fruit if you're lucky. Many airlines offer special diets with advance bookings and although there's no guarantee it meets your nutritional criteria, it may give you healthier choices compared to what everyone else is having.

Traveling domestic economy these days, it's probably best to eat before you leave, take your own snacks with you and decline the in-flight snack (you really will be better off without that mini chocolate bar, cookie, cake, or muffin, which on some airlines you have to pay for).

Our suggestions:

❏ Fresh fruit, soup, and salad items in airline lounges rather than white bread, cheese, cakes, and salami

❏ Small meals in-flight, rather than eating everything put in front of you

❏ Water to drink, wherever you are

❏ Dried fruit, nut bars, bananas, or apples that you have taken along yourself

Gluten-free eating out

Eating out on a gluten-free diet can be difficult, particularly as there is often gluten in items such as sauces, stock, dressings, and gravy. It is important that the restaurant understands your need for a meal that is completely free of gluten, and it may be a good idea to call beforehand to ensure that they can accommodate your needs.

You may have a local celiac society, which should be able to give you a list of recommended restaurants at which to eat, where you can be confident that they are able to provide you with a gluten-free meal. These are good places to start. Otherwise, you need to ask plenty of questions and remember that, if you are in doubt, you are best to leave it out!

Following are some tips to making low GI gluten-free meal choices when eating out.

- ❏ Plain grilled steak, chicken, or fish with corn on the cob, and salad or steamed vegetables

- ❏ Indian dahl with basmati rice

- ❏ Mexican tacos (if made with 100 percent corn tortillas) with beans, salad, avocado, salsa, and grated cheese

- ❏ Sushi filled with raw fish or avocado and cucumber (add pickled ginger and skip the soy sauce)

- ❏ Vietnamese rice paper rolls (but hold the dipping sauce unless you can check if it is gluten-free)

- ❏ Asian rice noodles stir-fried with vegetables, tofu, or shrimp, peanuts, cilantro, and lemon or lime juice (check the sauces)

- ❏ Mixed-bean, chickpea, or lentil salads (leave the dressing unless you can check it is gluten-free)

- ❏ Falafel (check they are gluten-free) with hummus and salad

For more on gluten-free eating, see pages 71–78.

Your eating out Q&A

What's the GI of a latte and cappuccino?

Most milky drinks will have a low GI and won't add too many calories either so long as you don't sweeten them with more than a teaspoon or so of sugar and say no to those flavored syrups lined up on the counter. In fact, a latte, cappuccino, or café au lait can be the perfect mid-morning snack and an easy way to help you get your two to three servings of dairy foods a day. Regular or skim milk has a low GI— a combination of the moderate glycemic effect of its sugar (lactose) plus milk protein, which forms a soft curd in the stomach and slows down stomach emptying. Regular full fat milk is high in saturated fat, but these days there's a wide range of reduced fat milks including low fat and skim types. If you prefer soy milk, make sure you opt for calcium fortified and reduced fat. Note that rice milk is not a suitable substitute; it has a high GI. Almond milk is a low-GI alternative and with fortification has about 75% of the calcium content of dairy milk.

How much milk are you getting with your coffee? Well, to some extent it depends on the cafe and where you buy it. But here are some standard definitions.

❑ A caffe latte is a single shot of espresso with steamed milk—approximately a 3:1 ratio of milk to coffee.

❑ A café au lait is similar except it is generally made with brewed coffee instead of espresso in a ratio of 1:1 milk to coffee.

❑ Cappuccino is traditionally equal parts espresso, steamed milk, and frothed milk.

How can I stick to low GI foods at parties, at work events, or during the holiday season?

For the right fuel, fitness, and stamina to make it through the nonstop demands of social occasions and the festive season, try these seven energy-boosting tips.

1. Make breakfast a priority

To nourish your body and sustain you through the morning, fire up your engine with low GI carbs. A good breakfast recharges your brain, speeds up your metabolism after an overnight fast, and reduces those feelings of stress.

2. Don't skip meals

Take a break to refuel at lunchtime to maintain energy levels right through the afternoon. Hold back on the high GI carbs to minimize that post-lunch energy dip. And take time over one main meal every day to make sure you aren't missing out on the vegetables you need.

3. Build your meals around low GI carbs

Food is the fuel needed to keep your body and brain energized. For daylong energy, fuel your body with low GI carbs that trickle glucose into your bloodstream. Use the 1, 2, 3 guide on page 16.

4. Try to be moderate

Pace yourself on the social merry-go-round by eating and drinking in moderation. If you are planning a big night out, don't starve yourself beforehand. All that does is reduce your metabolic rate. Have a light breakfast and lunch, and before you head off to the party eat a quick and easy low GI snack such as a sandwich made with grainy bread and a glass of low fat milk or a cup of yogurt and a dollop of fruit.

5. Be discerning with drinks

Make water your first choice. Ask for some routinely; chances are you'll drink it if it's in front of you. Go easy on the sugary drinks (they tend to bypass satiety mechanisms) and drink no more than one to three glasses of alcohol.

6. Move it

Cut holiday stress in its tracks. Exercise helps to relieve stress (it releases the "feel good" chemicals that negate energy and stress) and keeps your body strong. Get on your bike or into your sneakers and get that heart rate pumping for at least 20 minutes a day.

7. Get enough sleep

Get seven or eight hours sleep, so plan for as many early nights as you can.

Low GI
gluten-free eating

Gluten-free eating

If you have been diagnosed with celiac disease or gluten intolerance, a gluten-free diet is necessary for good health. In the absence of these conditions, there is no health benefit in avoiding gluten.

There is much more to a gluten-free lifestyle than focusing on foods you need to avoid. Eating well is the key to good health for everyone, and eating the right foods gives your body the fuel it needs to perform at its best and the energy to get through the day. It's also an important part of managing and preventing other long-term health problems, including diabetes, heart disease, cancer, and a range of digestive problems.

If you have celiac disease and need to follow a strict gluten-free diet, we suggest that you join a local celiac group and take advantage of the up-to-date and comprehensive information they provide for their members on shopping, cooking, and eating gluten-free. Recent research has also found that some people are sensitive to gluten yet not allergic (as in celiac disease). Symptoms include bloating, flatulence, and lethargy. Gluten-free diets have been found to be helpful.

While it is great to see an increasing range of ready-made gluten-free foods making life easier for those with celiac disease, unfortunately many of them are highly processed and some are high in fat and added sugar—two ingredients that are naturally gluten-free!

What is gluten?

Gluten is the protein found in the grains wheat, rye, barley, and triticale. Oats are frequently grown, harvested, milled, and processed alongside gluten-containing grains, so they may be contaminated with gluten. They also contain a gluten-like protein which some people with celiac disease react to. So, while research is ongoing, oats are currently not recommended for people with celiac disease (unless clearly marked as gluten-free).

Gluten-free diets also tend to have a high glycemic index (GI). This is because many low GI staples such as whole wheat kernel breads, pasta, barley, and oats are eliminated because they contain gluten. The gluten-free alternatives, due to their ingredients and processing methods, are often quickly digested and absorbed, raising blood glucose and insulin levels and leaving you feeling hungry and often low on energy a few hours after eating. What this means in practice is that many people following a gluten-free diet are rarely satisfied after meals and may feel hungry between meals, which can lead to overeating and weight gain.

In addition, adults and children on a gluten-free diet can miss out on the numerous health benefits of:

❑ Getting enough fiber

❑ Managing blood glucose levels with low GI foods.
(See the benefits of a low GI diet on page 4.)

Even on a wheat-free or gluten-free diet, you'll find that there are many low GI gluten-free foods you can enjoy in four of the five food groups:

❑ Virtually all fruits and vegetables

❑ Some whole kernel grains in the breads and cereals group

❑ Legumes of all types in the meat and alternatives group

❑ Milk and yogurt among the dairy foods

There are a number of gluten-free breads, breakfast cereals, snack foods, and pastas on the market. As not many have been GI tested, here are some guidelines for selecting lower GI options.

Bread
Most of the gluten-free breads tested, including rolls and wraps, have been found to have a high GI. But here is a tip: check out the ingredients list and opt for breads that include chickpea- or legume-based flours and psyllium. For example, we know that chapatis made with besan (chickpea flour) have a low GI. If you make your own bread, try adding buckwheat kernels, rice bran, and psyllium husks to lower the GI.

Breakfast cereals
Most gluten-free breakfast cereals, including rice, buckwheat, or millet puffs and flakes, have a moderate or high GI because they are refined, not whole-grain, foods.

But you can reduce the GI if you serve them with fruit and yogurt and a teaspoon or two of psyllium to boost the fiber. If you like cooked cereal, try quinoa porridge (made from whole quinoa grains) or make your own rice porridge (from a lower GI rice). Add psyllium husks and rice bran, along with fruit and low fat milk or yogurt.

Noodles and pasta
There are several low GI, gluten-free options available in both fresh and dried varieties:

❑ Buckwheat noodles

❑ Cellophane noodles, also known as mung bean noodles

❑ Rice noodles, made from ground or pounded rice flour

Most gluten-free pastas based on rice and corn tend to have moderate to high GI values. So opt for pastas made from legumes or soy—although they may be harder to find.

Whole cereal grains
Low GI cereal grains for those on a gluten-free diet include buckwheat, quinoa, and some varieties of rice and corn. Currently there are no published values for amaranth, sorghum, and teff. Millet has a high GI.

Rice
Rice can have a very high GI value or a moderate one, depending on the variety and its amylose content. Instant

and quick-cooking rices all tend to have a high GI. So, if you are a big rice eater, opt for the lower GI varieties with a higher amylose content such as basmati rice (GI = 58) or SunRice Low GI white or brown rice (GI = 54).

Brown rice is an extremely nutritious form of rice and contains several B-group vitamins, minerals, dietary fiber, and protein. The varieties tested to date tend to have a moderate or high GI (SunRice Low GI varieties excepted), so try to combine this nourishing food with low GI ingredients like lentils or beans, or even in combination with wild rice.

Wild rice (GI = 57) is not rice at all, but a type of grass seed. Arborio rice, used mainly in risotto, releases its starch during cooking and has a medium GI.

Legumes (beans)
Dried or canned legumes, including beans, chickpeas, and lentils, are among nature's lowest GI foods. They are high in fiber and packed with nutrients, providing protein, carbohydrate, B vitamins, folate, and minerals. Check canned varieties for gluten content.

When you add legumes to meals and snacks, you reduce the overall GI of your diet because your body digests them slowly. This is primarily because their starch breaks down relatively slowly (or incompletely) during cooking, and they contain tannins and enzyme inhibitors that also slow digestion. So make the most of beans, chickpeas, lentils, and whole and split dried peas.

Nuts

Although nuts are high in fat (averaging around 50 percent of their content), that fat is largely unsaturated, so they make a healthy substitute for snacks such as biscuits, cakes, pastries, potato chips, and chocolate. They also contain relatively little carbohydrate, so most do not have a GI value. Peanuts and cashews have very low GI values. Avoid the varieties that are salted and cooked in oil— choose raw and unsalted. Also be aware that dry-roasted nuts may contain gluten.

Chestnuts are quite different from other nuts in that they are low in fat and higher in carbohydrate. Naturally gluten-free, they have recently been found to have a low GI, which makes them a great low GI, high-fiber carbohydrate food.

Low fat dairy foods and calcium-enriched soy products

Low fat varieties of milk, yogurt, and ice cream, or calcium-enriched soy alternatives, provide you with sustained energy, boosting your calcium intake but not your saturated fat intake. Check the labels of yogurts, ice creams, and soy milks, as some contain wheat-based maltodextrins, which should be avoided.

Cheese is a good source of calcium, but it is a protein food, not a carbohydrate—its lactose is drawn off in the whey during production. This means that GI is not relevant to cheese. Although perfect for sandwich fillings, snacks, and toppings for gratin dishes, remember that cheese can also contribute a fair number of calories. Most cheese is around 30 percent fat, much of it saturated. Ricotta and cottage cheese are good low fat choices.

For more information about celiac disease and gluten intolerance plus more than 80 recipes, check out *The New Glucose Revolution Low GI Gluten-Free Eating Made Easy: The Essential Guide to the Glycemic Index and Gluten-Free Living.*

See page 274 for more help on gluten-free eating.

Sugars and
Sweeteners

Do you feel guilty every time you enjoy something sweet? Do you think diabetes equals no sugar? Join the club. Many people think that if something tastes good, it must be bad for them. And many people with diabetes, and even their doctors, mistakenly believe that sugar consumption is the most important explanation for high blood glucose readings.

While we now know that's not the case, old habits die hard. Traditionally, people with diabetes have been told to replace all sugar with an artificial sweetener and to drink diet soda. It's enough to make some people with diabetes turn their backs on all dietary advice.

But wanting something sweet is instinctive, and hard to ignore. It is part of our "hardwiring." In our hunter-gatherer past, fruits, berries, and honey were a major source of carbohydrate energy.

You'll be relieved to know that most diabetes organizations all around the world no longer advise strict avoidance of refined sugar or sugary foods. This is one of the happy spin-offs from research on the GI—recognition that both sugary foods and starchy foods raise your blood glucose.

Furthermore, dozens of studies indicate that moderate amounts of added sugar in diabetic diets (for example, 30–50 grams per day) does not result in either poor control or weight gain. Yes, a soft drink can be a concentrated source of calories, but so can a fruit juice or an alcoholic drink.

But a word of caution: there is increasing evidence that energy in liquid forms (both soft drinks and fruit juices) may sneak past the brain's appetite center. For example, if you give people 100 extra calories as solid jelly beans, they unconsciously compensate by consuming fewer calories over the rest of the day. But if you feed them 100 calories in a soda, fruit juice, beer, or other liquid, they don't reduce their intake much at all. Those extra calories can head straight for the waistline. In a recent study at Harvard University, the children who became overweight over time were the ones who were greater consumers of soft drinks and fruit juices.

You can enjoy refined or "added" sugar in moderation—for example, a smear of jelly on a sandwich, a teaspoon of sugar in coffee, a squeeze of honey on oatmeal, or a sugar-sweetened yogurt. Even the World Health Organization says "a moderate intake of sugar-rich foods can provide for a palatable and nutritious diet." So forget the guilt trip and allow yourself the pleasure of sweetness.

Should we be concerned about fructose?

One form of sugar, fructose or fruit sugar, has been hitting the headlines because of the alarmist view that it's "toxic" to our metabolism and should be consumed in minimal amounts. We don't agree and neither do the experts! Indeed, we believe that avoiding fructose could do more harm than good.

Fructose represents about half the natural sugars in fruit, vegetables, and grains. It is also one half of the sucrose molecule (that's the one in cane or refined sugar) and as much as 70 percent of the total sugars in honey.

Fructose has a low GI (equivalent to 20) and in normal quantities it contributes to better diabetes control and lower blood pressure.

In the United States, average fructose consumption is 55 grams per day (11 teaspoons) with the highest consumers eating 73 grams (15 teaspoons). Nutritional analysis of a typical low GI menu generates 70 grams of sugar per day, of which 25–30 grams would be fructose.

Can fructose contribute to weight gain?

Of course! Like all carbohydrates, it contains 4 calories per gram, yet that's a lot less than the calories in a gram of fat (9 calories per gram) or alcohol (7 calories per gram). Recent expert reviews of all available human research on fructose concluded that fructose does not cause weight gain when it is substituted for other carbohydrates in diets providing similar calories. Consuming fructose *at very high doses* (more than 100 grams or 20 teaspoons per day) that provides excess calories may modestly increase body weight, but this effect is most likely due to the extra calories rather than the fructose.

From an evolutionary perspective, fructose was an important component of intelligent primate diets. Our human ancestors adored sweet berries and honey and made sweet drinks using both honey and floral nectars. In the 1980s, we analyzed hundreds of traditional Aboriginal bushfoods, including sugarbag (bush honey) and dried bush fruits, such as the bush tomato *Solanum central*, which is 80 percent (by weight) sugar. In other parts of the world, apiculture, the art of raising bees, was widely practiced, even by the poor. Indeed at certain times in history, consumption of honey may well have rivaled our current consumption of refined sugar.

Strict avoidance of sugars and fructose reduces the enjoyment and quality of life for millions of people who enjoy a "spoonful of sugar." The take-home message is that a moderate consumption of fructose is compatible with a palatable and nutritious diet.

What about alternative sweeteners?

Alternatives to sugar are widely used by people with diabetes to sweeten drinks (tea and coffee) and foods (breakfast cereals); to sweeten recipes (for cakes and desserts); and in low-calorie commercial products (soft drinks, fruit punch, jams, gelatins, and yogurts).

They do give you sweetness with fewer calories, and usually with less effect on blood glucose levels, but there are differences between them.

Not all alternative sweeteners are the same—some have just as many calories as sugar; others have no calories at all; some are thousands (yes, thousands) of times sweeter than sugar; others are not very sweet at all. One thing they all have in common, however, is that they are more expensive than sugar.

There are lots of brands of sweeteners on the supermarket shelves, but essentially there are two main types:

❑ Nutritive sweeteners, and

❑ Nonnutritive sweeteners.

What's the difference?

Nutritive sweeteners

Nutritive sweeteners are simply those that provide some calories and, as the name suggests, nutrients. Sugar, for example, is a nutritive sweetener, but so are things like sorbitol and maltodextrin. They have differing effects on blood glucose levels.

Old-fashioned table sugar stands up well under scrutiny— it is the second sweetest after fructose, has only a moderate GI, is the best value for money, and is the easiest to use in cooking. And because it generally has a lower GI than the refined flour used in baking, it can actually lower the GI of many recipes! Less-refined sweeteners like raw sugar, honey, golden syrup, and pure (100%) maple syrup also provide small amounts of calcium, potassium, and magnesium.

The sugar alcohols, such as sorbitol, mannitol, and maltitol, are generally not as sweet as table sugar, provide fewer calories, and have less of an impact on blood glucose levels. To overcome their lack of sweet-ness, food manufacturers usually combine them with nonnutritive sweeteners to help keep the calorie count down and minimize the effect on blood glucose levels. This will be shown in the ingredients list on the food label.

The nutritive sweeteners such as sorbitol, mannitol, xylitol, and maltitol, and maltitol syrup, may have a laxative effect or cause gas or diarrhea if you consume them in large amounts. Foods that contain more than 10 grams per 100 grams of these alternative sweeteners, or more than 25 grams per 100 grams of sorbitol, isomalt, or polydextrose, carry warning statements about the possible laxative effect on their labels. These products can be a particular problem for children and adolescents, because of their smaller body size.

Used in sensible quantities, fructose certainly rivals table sugar as a good all-around sweetener. It stands out from the crowd, being nearly twice as sweet as sugar, providing the same number of calories, but having only one-third the GI. So you can use less fructose to achieve the same level of sweetness, and as a result, consume fewer calories and experience a much smaller rise in your blood glucose levels. Its main drawback is cost.

If you have read alarmist reports about fructose and blood fats and/or insulin resistance, remember that most of this research was on rats and mice fed excessive quantities of pure added fructose—more than someone with even the sweetest tooth could tolerate. There is no evidence that fructose has adverse effects in people with diabetes consuming normal quantities, e.g., less than 100 grams of added fructose per day.

What about Stevia and Monk Fruit?

Stevia has become popular with people seeking a more 'natural' alternative sweetener. Its natural reputation stems from the fact that it is derived from a sweet-tasting herb (*Stevia rebaudiana*), although stevia sweetener comes from a highly purified part of the plant (steviol glycosides). The leaves of the herb can be used as a sweetener themselves, and in the dried form less than 2 tablespoons of crushed leaves can replace the sweetness of about 1 cup of sugar. In commercial powdered products the steviol glycosides are usually combined with other substances to provide bulk or improve taste and texture. You can buy stevia in purified liquid and powder form and also in combination with other sugar replacers in tablet, powdered, and granulated form.

Like stevia, monk fruit (luo han guo), from Central Asia, is another natural alternative sweetener. The sweet extract of monk fruit, which is 200–300x sweeter than sugar, is usually combined with a dextrin or the sugar alcohol, erythritol, in commercial granulated products.

Both stevia and monk fruit sweetener are suitable for cooking. Both are virtually calorie free, tooth-friendly, and have no impact on blood glucose levels.

Nonnutritive sweeteners

Nonnutritive sweeteners (such as Equal, Splenda, or saccharin) are all much sweeter than table sugar and essentially have no effect on your blood glucose levels because most are used in such small quantities and are either not absorbed into or metabolized by the body. Because they are only used in minute amounts, the number of calories they provide is insignificant.

What's best to use for cooking?

The nonnutritive sweeteners that are made of protein molecules often break down when heated at high temperatures for long periods, thus losing their sweetness. For this reason, they are not always ideal for baking. The best nonnutritive sweeteners to cook with are Splenda, and saccharin, and to a lesser extent Equal Spoonful.

Are they safe?

As a group, nonnutritive sweeteners have been studied more thoroughly than any other type of food additive. Questions about the safety of saccharin were raised when it was first discovered over 125 years ago, and its effect on human health has been monitored ever since. The same is true of more recent sweeteners such as aspartame and sucralose. There is no convincing evidence so far that any of the nonnutritive sweeteners on the market have any negative effects on our health.

While the nonnutritive sweeteners available in North America are considered safe for everyone, some health professionals opt for caution and recommend that

---

Phenylketonuria and Aspartame

Food and beverages in the United States and Canada that contain aspartame must carry a warning for people with phenylketonuria. Phenylketonuria is a rare genetic disease, which is characterized by an inability of the body to utilize the essential amino acid, phenylalanine. About 1 in 10,000 newborn babies is affected with the condition. Managing this disease includes sticking to a low-protein diet, with particular emphasis on avoiding foods high in phenylalanine. As aspartame contains a significant amount of phenylalanine, it is not recommended for people with phenylketonuria.

---

pregnant women avoid saccharin and cyclamate. This is because both of them cross the placenta into the growing fetus and can also be found in breast milk.

Also, studies in rats have shown an increased risk of bladder cancer due to saccharin use and kidney disease due to cyclamate use. To put this in perspective, remember that saccharin and cyclamate were both used widely after World War II because there was a worldwide sugar shortage, and we did not see an increase in bladder or kidney cancer over that period. So it seems unlikely that either sweetener is a problem for pregnant women or those who are breastfeeding. However, some women still choose to avoid these two nonnutritive sweeteners.

Blends: the best of both worlds?

Splenda Sugar Blend for Baking is a blend of ordinary table sugar and sucralose, a nonnutritive sweetener. By adding sucralose to sugar, you get the best of both worlds: an intense sweetener with fewer calories, but the cooking properties of sugar. Its only downside is its cost—nearly three times that of table sugar.

The last word

Alternative sweeteners have been around for a very long time but have had little impact on the rate of obesity. In fact there is insufficient evidence to suggest that they benefit body weight, energy balance, appetite control, intake of carbohydrates, or cardiovascular risk factors.

If there are places in your diet where you are consuming large amounts of added sugar, you may benefit from replacing this with an alternative nonnutritive sweetener (see pages 214–221 for more detailed information on nutritive and nonnutritive sweeteners). For the rest of the time, just have a teaspoon or two of sugar and enjoy it.

GI values

Using the tables

These tables will help you put those low GI food choices into your shopping cart and onto your plate. Each entry lists an individual food and its GI value along with nutritional information for each food—fat (g), saturated fat (g), fiber (g), and sodium (mg). We also list the nominal serving size, the amount of carbohydrate per serving, and whether the food's GI is low, medium, or high.

A low GI value is 55 or less
A medium/moderate GI value is 56 to 69 inclusive
A high GI value is 70 or more

You can use the tables to:

❑ find the GI of your favorite foods

❑ compare carb-rich foods within a category (two types of bread or breakfast cereal for example)

❑ identify the best carbohydrate choices

❑ improve your diet by finding a low GI substitute for high GI foods

❑ put together a low GI meal

❑ find foods with a high GI but low GL

Each individual food appears alphabetically within a food category, like "Bread" or "Fruit." This makes it easy to compare the kinds of foods you eat every day and helps you see which high GI foods you could substitute with low GI versions.

The food categories are listed alphabetically, but if you need to find one quickly, check the category index on page 96. For instance, if you wanted to find the GI value of an apple, then you would look under the food category "Fruit." You could check the page number for "Fruit" in the category index.

The food categories used in the tables are:

❑ **Beans and legumes**—including baked beans, chickpeas, lentils, and split peas

❑ **Beverages**—including fruit and vegetable juices, soft drinks, flavored milk, and sport drinks

❑ **Bread**—including sliced white and whole grain bread, fruit breads, flatbreads, and crispbreads

❑ **Breakfast cereals**—including processed cereals, muesli, oats, and oatmeal

❑ **Cakes and muffins**—including other baked goods

❑ **Cereal grains**—including bulgur and barley

❑ **Cookies and crackers**

❑ **Dairy products**—including cheese, milk, yogurt, ice creams, and dairy desserts

❑ **Fruit**—including fresh, canned, and dried fruit (see *Beverages* for fruit juices)

❑ **Gluten-free products**

❑ **Meals, prepared/convenience**

- ❏ **Meat, seafood, eggs and protein**
- ❏ **Nutritional supplements**
- ❏ **Nuts and seeds**
- ❏ **Oils and dressings**
- ❏ **Pasta and noodles**
- ❏ **Rice**
- ❏ **Snack foods**—including chocolate, fruit bars, granola bars, and nuts
- ❏ **Soups**
- ❏ **Soy products**—including soy milk and soy yogurt
- ❏ **Spreads and sweeteners**—including sugars, honey, jam
- ❏ **Nutritive sweeteners**
- ❏ **Nonnutritive sweeteners**
- ❏ **Vegetables**—including green vegetables, salad vegetables and root vegetables (see *Beverages* for vegetable juices)
- ❏ **Weight management products**

In the tables you will sometimes see these symbols:
★ indicates that a food contains little or no carbohydrate. We have included these foods—like vegetables and protein-rich foods—because so many people ask us for their GI.

@ indicates that a food is part of the GI Symbol Program.
Foods with the GI symbol have had their GI tested
properly and are a healthy choice for their food
category.

To make a fair comparison, all foods have been tested using
an internationally standardized method. Gram for gram
of carbohydrates, the higher the GI, the higher the blood
glucose levels after consumption. If you can't find the GI
value for a food you regularly eat in these tables, check
out our website (www.glycemicindex.com). We maintain
an international database of published GI values that have
been tested by a reliable laboratory. Alternatively, please
write to the manufacturer and encourage them to have the
food tested by an accredited laboratory such as Sydney
University's Glycemic Index Research Service (SUGiRS).
In the meantime, choose a similar food from the tables as
a substitute.

The GI values in this book are correct at the time of
publication. However, the formulation of commercial
foods can change and the GI may change as well. You
can rely on foods showing the GI symbol. Although some
manufacturers include the GI on the nutritional label,
you would need to know that the testing was carried out
independently by an accredited laboratory.

Category index

BEANS & LEGUMES

FOOD	GI	LOW MED HIGH	SERVING SIZE
Baked beans, canned in tomato sauce, Heinz®	49	low	5 oz
Black beans, boiled	30	low	2¼ oz
Black-eyed beans, soaked, boiled	42	low	4¼ oz
Broad beans, frozen, reheated	63	med	3 oz
Butter beans, canned, drained	36	low	6 oz
Butter beans, dried, boiled	31	low	5¼ oz
Butter beans, soaked overnight, boiled 50 minutes	26	low	5¼ oz
Cannellini beans, canned, drained	31	low	5 oz
Chickpeas, canned, drained	38	low	5 oz
Chickpeas, canned in brine	40	low	4 oz
Chickpeas, dried, boiled	28	low	3 oz
Cranberry beans, canned, drained	41	low	2¼ oz
Four bean mix, canned, drained	37	low	3½ oz
Kidney beans, dark red, canned, drained	43	low	3½ oz
Kidney beans, red, canned, drained	36	low	6½ oz
Kidney beans, red, dried, boiled	28	low	3 oz
Kidney beans, red, soaked overnight, boiled 60 mins	51	low	3 oz
Lentils, brown, canned, drained	42	low	5¼ oz
Lentils, green, canned	48	low	4¾ oz
Lentils, green, dried, boiled	30	low	4½ oz
Lentils, red, dried, boiled	26	low	4½ oz
Lentils, red, split, boiled 25 mins	21	low	4½ oz

© part of GI symbol program   ★ little or no carbs

HOUSEHOLD MEASURE	CALORIES	FAT (g)	SATURATED FAT (g)	CARBO-HYDRATE (g)	FIBER (g)	SODIUM (mg)
½ cup	114	1	0	18	6	411
⅓ cup	86	0	0	15	6	1
⅔ cup	125	1	0	17	8	5
½ cup	60	0	0	7	3	7
1 cup	118	0	0	17	8	711
⅔ cup	120	1	0	17	8	11
⅔ cup	120	1	0	17	8	11
½ cup	127	0	0	14	9	213
⅔ cup	166	2	0	25	6	416
⅔ cup	123	2	0	16	5	288
½ cup	115	2	0	14	5	9
⅓ cup	92	0	0	17	2	1
½ cup	97	0	0	14	6	310
½ cup	98	1	0	14	6	304
¾ cup	161	1	0	19	10	495
½ cup	119	0	0	13	9	2
½ cup	119	0	0	13	9	2
1 cup	135	1	0	21	6	350
⅔ cup	87	0	0	13	4	419
⅔ cup	96	1	0	12	5	10
⅔ cup	96	1	0	12	5	10
⅔ cup	96	1	0	12	5	10

BEANS & LEGUMES

FOOD	GI	LOW MED HIGH	SERVING SIZE
Lima beans, baby, frozen, reheated	32	low	4 oz
Mung beans, boiled	39	low	5 oz
Peas, dried, boiled	22	low	6¼ oz
Peas, green, frozen, boiled	51	low	5½ oz
Pinto beans, canned, drained	45	low	4 oz
President's Choice® Blue Menu™ low fat 4-bean salad	13	low	3 oz
Refried pinto beans, canned, Casa Fiesta™	38	low	4 oz
Romano beans	46	low	5 oz
Soy beans, canned, drained	14	low	6 oz
Soy beans, dried, boiled	18	low	6 oz
Split peas, yellow, boiled 20 mins	32	low	6¼ oz
Split peas, yellow, dried, soaked overnight, boiled 55 mins	25	low	6¼ oz
White/navy beans, cooked, canned	38	low	2¼ oz
White/navy beans, dried, boiled	33	low	4 oz

ⓖ part of GI symbol program   ★ little or no carbs

HOUSEHOLD MEASURE	CALORIES	FAT (g)	SATURATED FAT (g)	CARBO-HYDRATE (g)	FIBER (g)	SODIUM (mg)
⅔ cup	126	1	0	15	10	9
⅔ cup	152	3	1	16	11	17
1 cup	118	1	0	13	7	16
1 cup	113	1	0	13	9	5
½ cup	103	1	0	18	5	353
⅓ cup	70	0	0	9	5	320
½ cup	112	1	0	20	3	338
½ cup	44	0	0	9	2	354
1 cup	169	9	1	5	8	629
1 cup	242	13	2	2	12	15
1 cup	118	1	0	13	7	16
1 cup	118	1	0	13	7	16
⅓ cup	74	0	0	13	3	291
⅔ cup	126	1	0	15	10	9

BEVERAGES

FOOD	GI	LOW MED HIGH	SERVING SIZE
Apple and Cherry juice, pure	43	low	8 fl oz
Apple and Mango juice, pure	47	low	8 fl oz
Apple and Pineapple juice	48	low	8 fl oz
Apple juice, filtered, pure	44	low	8 fl oz
Apple juice, Granny Smith, unsweetened	44	low	8 fl oz
Apple juice, no added sugar	40	low	8 fl oz
Apple juice with fiber	37	low	8 fl oz
Beer (4.6% alcohol)	66	med	12 fl oz
Campbell's, 100% vegetable juice	43	low	6 fl oz
Campbell's, tomato juice	33	low	12 fl oz
Campbell's V8 Splash, tropical blend fruit drink	47	low	8 fl oz
Carrot juice, freshly made	43	low	8 fl oz
Chocolate Daydream™ shake, fructose, Revival Soy®	33	low	8 fl oz
Chocolate Daydream™ shake, sucralose, Revival Soy®	25	low	8 fl oz
Chocolate-flavored milk	37	low	8 fl oz
Chocolate milkshake, commercial	21	low	16 fl oz
Coca-Cola®	53	low	12 fl oz
Cocoa with water	★		8 fl oz
Coffee, black	★		8 fl oz
Coffee, cappuccino	★		8 fl oz
Coffee, milk	★		8 fl oz
Cola, artificially sweetened	★		8 fl oz

⑥ part of GI symbol program   ★ little or no carbs

HOUSEHOLD MEASURE	CALORIES	FAT (g)	SATURATED FAT (g)	CARBO-HYDRATE (g)	FIBER (g)	SODIUM (mg)
1 cup	138	0	0	33	0	10
1 cup	126	0	0	33	2	8
1 cup	126	0	0	34	0	2
1 cup	130	0	0	30	0	8
1 cup	100	0	0	30	0	22
1 cup	100	0	0	28	0	11
1 cup	120	0	0	28	0	8
1 can	150	0	0	12	0	14
1 can	38	0	0	6	2	465
1 bottle	75	0	0	11	3	1125
1 cup	110	0	0	27	0	50
1 cup	71	0	0	14	2	118
1 cup	240	3	1	36	2	320
1 cup	120	3	1	7	2	320
1 cup	210	9	6	24	0	151
1 medium beverage	478	14	9	68	0	365
1 can	156	0	0	41	0	43
1 cup	6	0	0	0	0	13
1 cup	3	0	0	0	0	9
1 cup	55	3	2	4	0	42
1 cup	29	1	1	2	0	26
1 cup	2	0	0	0	0	32

BEVERAGES

FOOD	GI	LOW MED HIGH	SERVING SIZE
Cranberry juice cocktail	52	low	8 fl oz
Diet Coke®	★		8 fl oz
Diet dry ginger ale	★		8 fl oz
Diet ginger beer	★		8 fl oz
Diet lemonade	★		8 fl oz
Diet orange fruit drink	★		12 fl oz
Fanta® orange soft drink	68	med	8 fl oz
Fruit punch	67	med	8 fl oz
Grapefruit juice, unsweetened	48	low	8 fl oz
Hot Chocolate mix made with hot water, 1 pkt.	51	low	6 fl oz
Lemonade	54	low	8 fl oz
Lemonade, artificially sweetened	★		8 fl oz
Lemonade, Schweppes	54	low	12½ oz
Malted powder in full fat milk	45	low	8 fl oz
Mango smoothie	32	low	8 fl oz
Mineral water	★		8 fl oz
MonaVie E^{MV™}	52	low	8 fl oz
Nesquik® powder, Chocolate, in 2% fat milk	41	low	8 fl oz
Nesquik® powder, Strawberry, in 2% fat milk	35	low	8 fl oz
Orange juice, unsweetened, fresh	50	low	8 fl oz
Orange juice, unsweetened, from concentrate	53	low	8 fl oz

@ part of GI symbol program   ★ little or no carbs

HOUSEHOLD MEASURE	CALORIES	FAT (g)	SATURATED FAT (g)	CARBO-HYDRATE (g)	FIBER (g)	SODIUM (mg)
1 cup	134	0	0	34	0	6
1 cup	1	0	0	0	0	30
1 cup	3	0	0	0	0	20
1 cup	1	0	0	0	0	48
1 cup	2	0	0	0	0	14
1 can	11	0	0	3	0	30
1 cup	128	2	0	30	0	12
1 cup	120	0	0	29	0	25
1 cup	84	0	0	18	0	13
1 small cup	112	1	1	23	1	150
1 cup	104	0	0	28	0	42
1 cup	4	0	0	0	0	41
1 can	170	0	0	41	0	79
1 cup	278	6	4	30	0	206
1 bottle	122	1	0	30	0	28
1 cup	0	0	0	0	0	23
1 cup	160	0	0	40	0	20
1 cup	170	2	1	26	0	126
1 cup	170	2	1	26	0	118
1 cup	86	0	0	19	1	13
1 cup	86	0	0	19	1	13

BEVERAGES

FOOD	GI	LOW MED HIGH	SERVING SIZE
Pepsi Max	★		8 fl oz
Pineapple juice, unsweetened	46	low	8 fl oz
Pomegranate juice	53	low	8 fl oz
President's Choice® Blue Menu™ Oh Mega j orange juice	48	low	8 fl oz
President's Choice® Blue Menu™ Soy Beverage, Chocolate flavored	40	low	8 fl oz
President's Choice® Blue Menu™ Soy Beverage, Original flavored	15	low	8 fl oz
President's Choice® Blue Menu™ Soy Beverage, Vanilla flavored	28	low	8 fl oz
President's Choice® Blue Menu™ Tomato juice, low sodium	23	low	8 fl oz
Prune juice	43	low	8 fl oz
Rice milk, low fat	86	high	8 fl oz
Sambazon Açai Original Juice	24	low	8 fl oz
Smoothie, banana	30	low	8 fl oz
Smoothie, banana and strawberry, V8 Splash®	44	low	8 fl oz
Smoothie, fruit	35	low	8 fl oz
Smoothie, mango	32	low	8 fl oz
Soda water	★		8 fl oz
Sprite Zero lemonade	★		8 fl oz
Strawberry-flavored milk	37	low	8 fl oz
Tea, black	★		8 fl oz

@ part of GI symbol program   ★ little or no carbs

HOUSEHOLD MEASURE	CALORIES	FAT (g)	SATURATED FAT (g)	CARBO-HYDRATE (g)	FIBER (g)	SODIUM (mg)
1 cup	1	0	0	0	0	8
1 cup	104	0	0	24	0	2
1 cup	140	0	0	35	0	30
1 cup	130	0	0	30	0	25
1 cup	160	3	1	28	0	140
1 cup	90	3	1	9	0	150
1 cup	120	3	1	16	0	160
1 cup	45	0	0	7	2	310
1 cup	144	0	0	36	2	10
1 cup	122	2	0	27	0	88
1 cup	150	3.5	1	31	1	10
1 cup	215	7	5	26	2	77
1 cup	90	0	0	20	0	70
1 cup	203	7	5	28	2	73
1 cup	215	7	5	26	2	77
1 cup	0	0	0	0	0	61
1 cup	2	0	0	0	0	30
1 cup	188	8	5	22	0	96
1 cup	3	0	0	0	0	7

BEVERAGES

FOOD	GI	LOW MED HIGH	SERVING SIZE
Tea, white	★		8 fl oz
Tomato juice, no added sugar	38	low	8 fl oz
Tonic water, artificially sweetened	★		8 fl oz
Tropical blend fruit drink	47	low	8 fl oz
@ Ultra Lo-Gly Acai Blue	23	low	8 fl oz
@ Ultra Lo-Gly Mango Mojito	23	low	8 fl oz
@ Ultra Lo-Gly Pomegranate	19	low	8 fl oz
@ Ultra Lo-Gly Pomegranate Mojito	19	low	8 fl oz
Vegetable Juice	43	low	8 fl oz

@ part of GI symbol program   ★ little or no carbs

HOUSEHOLD MEASURE	CALORIES	FAT (g)	SATURATED FAT (g)	CARBO-HYDRATE (g)	FIBER (g)	SODIUM (mg)
1 cup	16	1	1	1	0	16
1 cup	57	0	0	11	1	753
1 cup	0	0	0	0	0	0
1 cup	84	0	0	20	0	51
1 cup	35	0	0	9	0	10
1 cup	25	0	0	7	0	10
1 cup	35	0	0	8	0	10
1 cup	30	0	0	8	0	10
1 cup	51	0	0	10	2	420

BREAD

FOOD	GI	LOW MED HIGH	SERVING SIZE
3 Grain bread, sprouted grains	55	low	1½ oz
9 Grain muffin	43	low	1 oz
9 Grain original bread	39	low	1¼ oz
100% whole grain bread	51	low	1 oz
Apricot fruit bread	56	med	1½ oz
Bagel, white	72	high	3 oz
Baguette, traditional French bread	77	high	2 oz
Black rye bread	76	high	1½ oz
Bread roll, white	71	high	1 oz
Bread roll, whole wheat	70	high	1¼ oz
COBS Bread Higher-Fiber Low GI White Bread, unsliced	46	low	2 oz
Continental fruit bread	47	low	¾ oz
Corn tortilla	52	low	1 oz
Country life grain bread	61	med	2½ oz
Croissant, plain	67	med	1 oz
Crumpet	69	med	1¼ oz
@ EnerGI white sandwich bread	58	med	1¼ oz
Flaxseed and soy bread	55	low	3 oz
Hamburger bun, white	61	med	1 oz
Homemade white bread	70	high	1¼ oz
Hot dog roll, white	68	med	1½ oz
Italian bread	73	high	1¼ oz

@ part of GI symbol program   ★ little or no carbs

HOUSEHOLD MEASURE	CALORIES	FAT (g)	SATURATED FAT (g)	CARBO-HYDRATE (g)	FIBER (g)	SODIUM (mg)
1 slice	120	2	0	17	3	200
1 muffin	79	2	0	11	2	86
1 slice	69	2	0	13	2	167
1 slice	90	2	0	11	4	120
1 thick slice	116	0	0	24	2	124
1 whole	185	0	0	43	1	152
2 slices	162	1	0	31	1	362
1 slice	98	1	0	18	3	252
½ large (4-inch diameter)	97	1	0	17	1	188
½ large (4-inch diameter)	99	1	0	17	2	202
2 slices	170	0.5	0	38	6	390
1 slice	65	1	0	12	1	51
1 tortilla	74	1	0	14	2	54
2 slices	180	2	0	28	5	377
½ average	140	8	4	13	1	126
1 round	78	0	0	16	1	389
1 slice	93	1	0	17	2	162
2 slices	230	8	1	26	6	364
½ large (4-inch diameter)	97	1	0	18	1	188
1 thin slice	87	0	0	18	1	1
1 roll	120	2	0	22	1	206
1 slice	98	1	0	18	1	204

BREAD

FOOD	GI	LOW MED HIGH	SERVING SIZE
Kaiser roll, white	73	high	1 oz
Lebanese bread, white	75	high	1 oz
Light rye bread	68	med	1 oz
Melba toast, plain	70	high	½ oz
Multigrain sandwich bread	65	med	1 oz
Natural Ovens English Muffin™ bread	77	high	1 oz
Natural Ovens Happiness™, cinnamon, raisin, pecan bread	63	med	1 oz
Natural Ovens Hunger Filler™, whole grain bread	59	med	1 oz
Organic stoneground whole wheat sourdough bread	59	med	1¼ oz
Pita bread, white	57	med	1¼ oz
Pita, white, mini	68	med	1 oz
President's Choice® Blue Menu™ tortillas, flax	53	low	2 oz
President's Choice® Blue Menu™ Whole Grain English muffins	51	low	2 oz
President's Choice® Blue Menu™ Whole Grain Multi-Grain Flax Bagel	58	med	2 oz
President's Choice® Blue Menu™ Whole Grain Multi-Grain English Muffin	45	low	2 oz

@ part of GI symbol program   ★ little or no carbs

HOUSEHOLD MEASURE	CALORIES	FAT (g)	SATURATED FAT (g)	CARBO-HYDRATE (g)	FIBER (g)	SODIUM (mg)
¼ roll	77	1	0	15	1	161
½ medium (6- or 7-inch diameter)	98	1	0	19	1	158
¾ slice	82	1	0	14	2	176
1 slice	59	1	0	11	1	104
1 slice	77	1	0	14	1	135
1 slice	90	1	0	15	1	115
1 slice	90	2	0	12	3	90
1 slice	90	2	0	11	4	100
1 slice	95	1	0	17	1	218
½ medium (6- or 7-inch diameter)	98	1	0	17	1	158
1 pita	82	0	0	16	1	161
1 tortilla	140	5	1	29	3	480
1 muffin	140	3	0	20	3	130
1 bagel	170	3	1	28	5	200
1 muffin	140	3	0	20	3	130

BREAD

FOOD	GI	LOW MED HIGH	SERVING SIZE
President's Choice® Blue Menu™ Whole Wheat Soy bread	45	low	3 oz
Pumpernickel bread	50	low	1 oz
Raisin toast	63	med	1 oz
Rye bread, whole grain	58	med	1 oz
Sourdough rye bread	48	low	1¼ oz
Sourdough wheat bread	54	low	1 oz
Sourdough white bread	79	high	1 oz
Spelt multi-grain bread	54	low	1¼ oz
Stuffing, bread	74	high	2¾ oz
Taco shell	68	high	1 oz
Traditional sourdough bread	58	med	3 oz
Tortilla, reduced carbohydrate	51	low	1 oz
Turkish bread, white	87	high	3 oz
White bread, regular, sliced	71	high	1 oz
White bread, high fiber, low GI Baker's Delight	52	low	1¼ oz
White Vienna bread	66	med	1½ oz
Whole grain rye bread	58	med	1 oz
Whole wheat block loaf	71	high	2½ oz
Whole wheat sandwich bread	71	high	1 oz
Whole wheat country grain bread	53	low	2½ oz
Wonder White®	80	high	1 oz

@ part of GI symbol program ★ little or no carbs

HOUSEHOLD MEASURE	CALORIES	FAT (g)	SATURATED FAT (g)	CARBO-HYDRATE (g)	FIBER (g)	SODIUM (mg)
2 slices	210	3	1	27	7	240
1 slice	74	0	0	14	3	226
1 slice	90	1	0	17	1	74
1 slice	73	1	0	12	2	187
1 slice	96	1	0	18	2	211
1 slice	62	1	0	11	1	134
1 slice	81	0	0	16	1	174
1 slice	85	1	0	14	3	188
½ cup	152	7	2	17	2	410
1 large or 2 small	98	4	1	13	1	82
2 slices	218	1	0	42	2	451
1 tortilla	60	2	0	7	8	49
2 slices	197	2	0	40	2	425
1 slice	69	1	0	13	1	143
1 slice	86	1	0	15	4	218
2 slices	117	1	0	23	1	250
1 slice	83	1	0	15	2	211
2 slices	164	2	0	27	1	368
1 slice	75	1	0	12	2	135
2 slices	178	2	0	28	5	372
1 slice	69	1	0	12	1	128

BREAKFAST CEREALS

FOOD	GI	LOW MED HIGH	SERVING SIZE
All-Bran™, Kellogg's®	50	low	1 oz
All-Bran® Complete Wheat Flakes, Kellogg's®	60	med	1 oz
All-Bran® Bran Buds, Kellogg's®	58	med	1 oz
belVita Breakfast Biscuits, Cranberry	40	low	1½ oz
belVita Breakfast Biscuits, Crunchy Oats	54	low	1½ oz
belVita Breakfast Biscuits, Fruit & Fiber	47	low	1½ oz
belVita Breakfast Biscuits, Honey & Nut with Chocolate Chips	46	low	1½ oz
belVita Breakfast Biscuits, Milk & Cereal	45	low	1½ oz
Bran Flakes, Kellogg's®	74	high	¾ oz
Cheerios™, General Mills	74	high	1 oz
Coco Pops®, Kellogg's®	80	high	1 oz
Corn Flakes™, Kellogg's®	80	high	1 oz
Cream of Wheat™, Instant	74	high	6 oz
Cream of Wheat™	66	med	6 oz
Crispix™, Kellogg's®	87	high	1 oz
Froot Loops®, Kellogg's®	69	med	¾ oz
Frosted Flakes®, Kellogg's®	55	low	¾ oz
Gluten-free muesli	39	low	1½ oz
Golden Grahams™, General Mills	71	high	1 oz
Grape-nuts™, Post	71	high	8 oz

@ part of GI symbol program   ★ little or no carbs

HOUSEHOLD MEASURE	CALORIES	FAT (g)	SATURATED FAT (g)	CARBO-HYDRATE (g)	FIBER (g)	SODIUM (mg)
½ cup	80	1	0	23	10	80
⅔ cup	107	1	0	21	4	99
⅓ cup	70	1	0	24	13	200
4 biscuits	200	7	2	34	3	150
4 biscuits	230	8	2	34	2.5	276
4 biscuits	226	8	2	32	3	76
4 biscuits	234	9	2	34	2	177
4 biscuits	230	8	2	35	2	214
½ cup	72	0	0	14	3	66
1 cup	110	2	0	21	2	250
1 cup	120	0	0	27	3	105
1 cup	100	0	0	24	1	200
1 cup	149	1	0	33	1	10
1 cup	131	1	0	29	1	8
1 cup	110	0	0	25	0	210
½ cup	78	0	0	17	1	94
½ cup	75	0	0	17	1	141
½ cup	183	11	5	13	7	12
¾ cup	120	1	0	25	1	280
1 cup	200	1	0	48	7	290

BREAKFAST CEREALS

FOOD	GI	LOW MED HIGH	SERVING SIZE
Grape-nuts™ Flakes, Post	80	high	1.1 oz
Hi-Bran Weet-Bix®, regular	61	med	1 oz
Honey Smacks®, Kellogg's®	71	high	1 oz
Just Right®, Kellogg's®	60	med	1½ oz
Kashi® 7 Whole Grain Puffs	65	med	0.7 oz
Life™, Quaker Oats	66	med	1 oz
Muesli, gluten and wheat free with psyllium	50	low	1½ oz
Muesli, mixed berry & apple	64	med	1½ oz
Muesli, Natural	40	low	1 oz
Muesli, Swiss Formula	56	med	1 oz
Muesli, yeast and wheat free	45	low	1½ oz
Oat bran, raw, unprocessed	55	low	1 oz
Oats, rolled, raw	55	low	1 oz
Oatmeal, multigrain, dry pkt, made with water	55	low	1 oz
Oatmeal, instant, made with water	83	high	6 oz
Oatmeal, made from steel-cut oats with water	52	low	6 oz
Oatmeal, regular, made from oats with water	58	med	6 oz
President's Choice® Blue Menu™ Bran Flakes	65	med	1 oz
President's Choice® Blue Menu™ Fiber-First, multi-bran cereal	55	low	1 oz

Ⓖ part of GI symbol program   ★ little or no carbs

HOUSEHOLD MEASURE	CALORIES	FAT (g)	SATURATED FAT (g)	CARBO-HYDRATE (g)	FIBER (g)	SODIUM (mg)
⅓ cup	110	1	0	24	3	120
1½ biscuits	107	2	1	17	6	122
¾ cup	104	1	0	23	1	50
¾ cup	153	1	0	32	2	253
1 cup	70	1	0	14	1	0
¾ cup	120	2	0	24	2	160
½ cup	183	11	5	13	7	12
½ cup	144	2	0	30	3	98
¼ cup	106	3	0	16	3	4
⅓ cup	110	2	0	18	3	33
½ cup	163	10	5	13	4	2
⅓ cup	114	2	1	17	3	3
⅓ cup	74	2	0	15	5	1
⅓ cup	96	1	0	17	3	1
¾ cup	101	3	0	18	3	0
¾ cup	101	3	0	18	3	0
¾ cup	101	3	0	18	3	0
¾ cup	110	1	0	24	5	190
½ cup	110	1	0	23	13	270

BREAKFAST CEREALS

FOOD	GI	LOW MED HIGH	SERVING SIZE
President's Choice® Blue Menu™ Granola Clusters, original, low-fat	63	med	2 oz
President's Choice® Blue Menu™ Granola Clusters, Raisin Almond, low-fat	70	high	2 oz
President's Choice® Blue Menu™ Omega-3 Granola Cereal	43	low	2 oz
President's Choice® Blue Menu™ Steel-Cut Oats	51	low	1¼ oz
Puffed buckwheat	65	med	¾ oz
Puffed Wheat, Quaker Oats	80	med	1 oz
Quick oats porridge	80	high	¾ oz
Quick oats	65	med	6 oz
Raisin Bran™, Kellogg's®	61	med	1 oz
Rice Krispies™, Kellogg's®	82	high	1.2 oz
Semolina, cooked	55	low	¾ oz
Shredded Wheat™, Post	83	high	1.6 oz
Special K™, Kellogg's®	69	med	1.1 oz
Total™, General Mills	76	high	1 oz
Weetabix™	74	high	1 oz

@ part of GI symbol program   ★ little or no carbs

HOUSEHOLD MEASURE	CALORIES	FAT (g)	SATURATED FAT (g)	CARBO-HYDRATE (g)	FIBER (g)	SODIUM (mg)
⅔ cup	220	3	1	40	4	55
⅔ cup	220	3	1	40	3	50
⅔ cup	230	6	1	37	5	65
¼ cup	150	2	0	29	4	0
½ cup	67	1	0	15	1	0
1 cup	102	1	0	21	3	1
⅔ cup	74	0	0	15	1	1
1 packet	100	2	0	19	3	80
½ cup	95	1	0	23	4	175
1¼ cups	120	0	0	29	0	320
½ cup	77	0	0	17	1	144
2 biscuits	160	1	0	37	6	0
1 cup	120	1	0	22	3	220
¾ cup	100	1	0	23	3	190
2 biscuits	130	1	0	28	4	135

CAKES & MUFFINS

FOOD	GI	LOW MED HIGH	SERVING SIZE
9 Grain muffin	43	low	I oz
Angel food cake	67	med	I oz
Apple berry crumble, commercially made	41	low	3½ oz
Apple muffin, homemade	46	low	1½ oz
Apple, oat, raisin muffin	54	low	1½ oz
Apricot, coconut and honey muffin	60	med	1½ oz
Banana, oat and honey muffin	65	med	1½ oz
Banana cake, homemade	51	low	1½ oz
Blueberry muffin	59	med	1½ oz
Blueberry muffin, commercially made	59	med	1½ oz
Bran muffin, commercially made	60	med	1½ oz
Carrot cake, commercially made	38	low	I oz
Carrot muffin, commercially made	62	med	1½ oz
Chocolate cake, made from packet mix with frosting, Betty Crocker®	38	low	I oz
Chocolate muffin	53	low	1½ oz
Chocolate butterscotch muffin	53	low	1½ oz

@ part of GI symbol program   ★ little or no carbs

HOUSEHOLD MEASURE	CALORIES	FAT (g)	SATURATED FAT (g)	CARBO-HYDRATE (g)	FIBER (g)	SODIUM (mg)
1 muffin	79	2	0	11	2	86
1 small piece (⅛ of a 10-inch cake)	77	1	0	15	0	137
1 serving	300	15	6	40	2	3
⅓ large	129	6	1	17	0	150
1 med. muffin	277	6	2	36	2	290
1 med. muffin	248	11	3	34	1	280
1 muffin	114	5	2	17	2	197
1 thin slice (⅛ of a 10-inch cake)	138	7	2	17	1	210
1 muffin	167	8	2	22	1	134
⅓ large	127	6	1	17	0	150
¾ average (2¾-inch diameter)	120	5	2	16	2	207
1 small piece	103	6	2	12	1	158
⅓ large	127	6	1	17	0	150
1 small piece (1/12 of a 6 x 2½ x 2½-inch cake)	110	6	3	14	0	91
½ medium (2¾-inch diameter)	150	7	1	18	1	93
1 med. muffin	302	18	4	31	1	146

CAKES & MUFFINS

FOOD	GI	LOW MED HIGH	SERVING SIZE
Croissant, plain	67	med	1 oz
Crumpet, white	69	med	1½ oz
Cupcake, strawberry-iced	73	high	1 oz
Double chocolate muffin	46	low	1½ oz
Doughnut, cinnamon sugar	75	high	1½ oz
Doughnut, commercially made	75	high	1½ oz
Egg custard	35	low	4 oz
Macaroons, coconut	32	low	1 oz
Oatmeal muffin, made from mix	69	med	1½ oz
Pancakes, buckwheat, gluten-free, packet mix	102	high	¾ oz
Pancakes, homemade	66	med	3 oz
Pancakes, prepared from mix (6-inch diameter)	67	med	2 oz
Pastry, puff	56	med	1 oz
Pound cake, Sara Lee®	54	low	1 oz
Scones, plain, made from packet mix	92	high	1 oz
Sponge cake, plain, unfilled	46	low	1 oz
Vanilla cake, made from packet mix with vanilla frosting, Betty Crocker®	42	low	1½ oz
Waffle, plain	76	high	1¼ oz
Waffle, toasted	76	high	1¼ oz

@ part of GI symbol program   ★ little or no carbs

HOUSEHOLD MEASURE	CALORIES	FAT (g)	SATURATED FAT (g)	CARBO-HYDRATE (g)	FIBER (g)	SODIUM (mg)
½ average	140	8	4	13	1	126
1 round	86	0	0	18	1	425
⅓ cupcake	84	2	1	15	0	91
1 muffin	187	9	2	24	1	117
1 small	168	9	4	18	1	171
1 doughnut	192	10	3	22	1	181
½ cup	117	4	2	15	0	109
1 cookie	115	4	3	22	1	70
1 muffin	129	6	1	17	2	150
1 small	67	0	0	15	1	95
2 pancakes	145	5	2	20	1	24
1 medium	143	7	3	18	1	111
⅛ sheet	171	12	2	15	1	77
1 small slice	109	6	3	14	0	111
1 small	110	3	1	17	1	182
1 slice (3-inch diameter)	72	1	0	14	0	60
1 thin slice (¹⁄₂₄ of a 10-inch cake)	151	7	2	19	0	150
1 square	141	7	3	16	1	335
1 square	141	7	3	16	1	335

CEREAL GRAINS

FOOD	GI	LOW MED HIGH	SERVING SIZE
Barley, pearled, boiled	25	low	2 oz
Buckwheat, boiled	54	low	3 oz
Bulgur, cracked wheat	48	low	3 oz
Millet, boiled	71	high	2½ oz
Polenta (cornmeal), boiled	68	med	6¾ oz
Quinoa, boiled	53	low	3½ oz
Rye, whole kernels	34	low	1 oz
Semolina, cooked	55	low	6 oz
Whole-wheat kernels, boiled	41	low	4 oz

@ part of GI symbol program   ★ little or no carbs

HOUSEHOLD MEASURE	CALORIES	FAT (g)	SATURATED FAT (g)	CARBO-HYDRATE (g)	FIBER (g)	SODIUM (mg)
⅓ cup	74	0	0	14	2	9
½ cup	89	1	0	17	1	4
⅓ cup	85	0	0	15	4	9
½ cup	83	1	0	16	0	1
¾ cup	46	0	0	16	1	0
½ cup	84	2	0	15	2	1
2 tbsp	67	1	0	14	3	1
¾ cup	65	0	0	13	1	0
½ cup	79	0	0	16	2	0

COOKIES & CRACKERS

FOOD	GI	LOW MED HIGH	SERVING SIZE
Breton wheat crackers	67	med	1 oz
Chocolate chip cookies	43	low	1 oz
Corn Thins, puffed corn cakes, gluten-free	87	high	1 oz
Digestives, plain	62	med	¾ oz
Highland Oatcakes, Walker's	57	med	1 oz
Kavli Norwegian crispbread	71	high	¾ oz
Macaroons, coconut	32	low	1 oz
Milk Arrowroot	69	med	¾ oz
Oatmeal cookies	54	low	¾ oz
Premium Soda Crackers	74	high	1 oz
President's Choice® Blue Menu™ Ancient Grains Snack Crackers	65	med	¾ oz
Puffed crispbread	81	high	1 oz
Puffed Rice Cakes, white	82	high	¾ oz
Rice cracker, plain	91	high	½ oz
Rich tea biscuits	55	low	¾ oz
Rye crispbread	63	med	1 oz
Ryvita® Fruit Crunch crispbread	66	med	½ oz
Ryvita® Original Rye crispbread	69	med	¾ oz
ⓖ Ryvita® Pumpkin Seeds and Oats crispbread	48	low	1 oz
Ryvita® Sesame Rye crispbread	64	med	¾ oz
ⓖ Ryvita® Sunflower Seeds and Oats crispbread	48	low	1 oz
Shortbread biscuits, plain	64	med	1 oz

HOUSEHOLD MEASURE	CALORIES	FAT (g)	SATURATED FAT (g)	CARBOHYDRATE (g)	FIBER (g)	SODIUM (mg)
7 crackers	118	5	2	14	1	279
2 cookies	137	7	2	18	1	98
4 slices	89	1	0	16	2	60
1½ cookies	110	5	2	15	1	154
2 oatcakes	110	5	2	13	1	160
4 crackers	68	1	0	14	3	70
1 cookie	115	4	3	22	1	70
2 cookies	77	2	1	13	1	47
2 cookies	103	5	3	14	1	141
3 crackers	80	3	1	21	1	304
10 crackers	80	2	0	12	2	160
3 crispbreads	95	1	0	18	1	137
2 rice cakes	75	1	0	15	1	1
8 crackers	60	1	0	11	0	78
3 cookies	111	4	2	18	1	116
3 crispbreads	70	0	0	28	5	75
1 crispbread	57	1	0	8	2	0
2 crispbreads	64	0	0	10	3	0
2 crispbreads	90	2	0	10	4	0
2 crispbreads	62	0	0	9	4	0
2 crispbreads	82	2	0	9	4	0
2 cookies	119	6	3	15	1	110

COOKIES & CRACKERS

FOOD	GI	LOW MED HIGH	SERVING SIZE
Shredded Wheat cookies	62	med	¾ oz
Spicy Apple fruit cookies (97% fat free)	45	low	1 oz
Stoned Wheat Thins	67	med	1 oz
Vanilla wafer cookies, plain	77	high	1 oz
Water cracker	63	med	1 oz
Wheat cracker, plain	67	med	1 oz

@ part of GI symbol program   ★ little or no carbs

HOUSEHOLD MEASURE	CALORIES	FAT (g)	SATURATED FAT (g)	CARBO-HYDRATE (g)	FIBER (g)	SODIUM (mg)
2 cookies	102	4	2	15	1	94
1 cookie	84	1	0	16	3	73
10 crackers	130	6	2	19	1	226
2 cookies	132	1	1	16	0	17
7 crackers	94	2	1	15	1	125
3 crackers	124	4	2	18	1	181

DAIRY PRODUCTS: CHEESES

FOOD	GI	LOW MED HIGH	SERVING SIZE
Brie	★		1 oz
Camembert	★		1 oz
Cheddar	★		1 oz
Cheddar, 25% reduced fat	★		1 oz
Cheddar, 50% reduced fat	★		1 oz
Cheddar, low fat	★		1 oz
Cheddar, reduced salt	★		1 oz
Cheese spread, cheddar	★		1 oz
Cheese spread, cheddar, reduced fat	★		1 oz
Cottage cheese	★		1 oz
Cottage cheese, low fat	★		1 oz
Cream cheese	★		1 oz
Cream cheese dip	★		1 oz
Cream cheese, reduced fat	★		1 oz
Feta	★		1 oz
Feta, low salt	★		1 oz
Feta, reduced fat	★		1 oz
Mozzarella	★		1 oz
Mozzarella, reduced fat	★		1 oz
Parmesan	★		1 oz
Ricotta	★		1 oz
Ricotta, reduced fat	★		1 oz
Soy cheese	★		1 oz

@ part of GI symbol program   ★ little or no carbs

HOUSEHOLD MEASURE	CALORIES	FAT (g)	SATURATED FAT (g)	CARBO-HYDRATE (g)	FIBER (g)	SODIUM (mg)
2 tbsp	102	9	6	0	0	182
2 tbsp	93	8	5	0	0	195
1 slice	122	10	7	0	0	197
1 slice	99	7	5	0	0	216
1 slice	80	5	3	0	0	207
1 slice	61	2	1	0	0	198
1 slice	123	11	7	0	0	111
1½ tbsp	87	7	5	1	0	435
1½ tbsp	72	5	3	2	0	480
2 tbsp	37	2	1	1	0	95
2 tbsp	27	0	0	1	0	39
1½ tbsp	102	10	6	1	0	126
1½ tbsp	76	7	4	3	0	204
1½ tbsp	58	5	3	1	0	102
2 tbsp	84	7	5	0	0	321
2 tbsp	113	10	7	0	0	66
2 tbsp	70	4	3	0	0	330
1 slice	91	7	4	0	0	113
1 slice	86	5	4	0	0	174
⅓ cup	133	10	6	0	0	432
2 tbsp	44	3	2	0	0	59
2 tbsp	38	3	2	0	0	56
1 slice	95	8	1	0	0	180

DAIRY PRODUCTS: ICE CREAM, CUSTARDS, PUDDINGS & DESSERTS

FOOD	GI	LOW MED HIGH	SERVING SIZE
Chocolate pudding, instant, made from packet with full fat milk	47	low	4½ oz
Chocolate shake, low fat chocolate soft serve with skim milk and malted milk powder	21	low	10 fl oz
Custard, homemade from milk, wheat starch and sugar	43	low	2 oz
Custard, low fat	38	low	4 fl oz
Gelato, sucrose-free, chocolate	37	low	2 oz
Gelato, sucrose-free, vanilla	39	low	2 oz
Ice cream, light creamy low fat, chocolate	27	low	2½ fl oz
Ice cream, light creamy low fat, English toffee	27	low	2½ fl oz
Ice cream, light creamy low fat, mango	30	low	2½ fl oz
Ice cream, light creamy low fat, vanilla	36	low	2½ fl oz
Ice cream, low carbohydrate, chocolate	32	low	3½ fl oz
Ice cream, regular, full fat, average	61	med	2½ fl oz
Low fat chocolate soft serve ice cream	24	low	2 oz
Low fat chocolate soft serve eaten with a plain cone	44	low	4 oz
Low fat chocolate soft serve eaten with a waffle cone	55	low	4 oz

@ part of GI symbol program   ★ little or no carbs

HOUSEHOLD MEASURE	CALORIES	FAT (g)	SATURATED FAT (g)	CARBO-HYDRATE (g)	FIBER (g)	SODIUM (mg)
⅙ packet	133	4	3	20	0	240
1 large cup	242	4	2	38	0	160
¼ cup	83	2	1	14	0	29
½ cup	102	1	1	18	0	59
1 scoop	84	3	2	14	0	34
1 scoop	76	2	1	14	0	34
1½ scoops	104	1	1	16	0	35
1½ scoops	74	1	1	14	1	30
1½ scoops	72	1	1	13	1	25
1½ scoops	93	1	1	17	1	38
2 scoops	61	2	1	5	5	44
1½ scoops	138	8	5	15	0	44
1 scoop	51	0	0	9	0	28
1 cone	108	2	1	20	1	53
1 cone	158	2	1	28	1	53

DAIRY PRODUCTS: ICE CREAM, CUSTARDS, PUDDINGS & DESSERTS

FOOD	GI	LOW MED HIGH	SERVING SIZE
President's Choice® Blue Menu™ Frozen yogurt, Mochaccino	51	low	4 fl oz
President's Choice® Blue Menu™ Frozen yogurt, Strawberry Banana	55	low	4 fl oz
President's Choice® Blue Menu™ Frozen yogurt, Vanilla	46	low	4 fl oz
Tapioca pudding, boiled, with milk	81	high	4 oz
Vanilla frozen yogurt	46	low	2½ oz
Vanilla pudding, instant, made from packet mix with full fat milk	40	low	3 oz
Wild Berry, non-dairy, frozen fruit dessert	59	med	1¾ fl oz

@ part of GI symbol program   ★ little or no carbs

HOUSEHOLD MEASURE	CALORIES	FAT (g)	SATURATED FAT (g)	CARBO-HYDRATE (g)	FIBER (g)	SODIUM (mg)
½ cup	120	2	1	21	0	65
½ cup	110	2	1	20	0	60
½ cup	110	2	1	21	0	65
½ cup	125	4	2	18	0	57
½ cup	114	4	2	17	0	63
⅛ packet prepared	103	3	2	15	0	190
1 scoop	48	0	0	12	0	10

DAIRY PRODUCTS: MILK & ALTERNATIVES

FOOD	GI	LOW MED HIGH	SERVING SIZE
Blue Diamond Refrigerated Unsweetened Vanilla Breeze (almond beverage)	23	low	8 fl oz
Blue Diamond Unsweetened Chocolate Breeze (almond beverage)	23	low	8 fl oz
Blue Diamond Unsweetened Original Breeze (almond beverage)	23	low	8 fl oz
Blue Diamond Unsweetened Vanilla Breeze (almond beverage)	23	low	8 fl oz
Chocolate-flavored, low fat milk	27	low	8 fl oz
Chocolate-flavored milk	37	low	5¼ fl oz
Condensed milk, sweetened, full fat	61	med	1 oz
Milk, whole (3.25%)	27–31	low	8 fl oz
Milk, low fat (1%)	20–30	low	8 fl oz
Milk, reduced fat (2%)	20–30	low	8 fl oz
Milk with omega-3	27	low	8 fl oz
Mocha-flavored, low fat milk	27	low	8 fl oz
Mocha-flavored milk, whole	32	low	8 fl oz
Probiotic fermented milk drink with *Lactobacillus casei*	46	low	2¼ fl oz
Skim milk, <1% fat	20–34	low	8 fl oz
Strawberry-flavored milk	37	low	6 fl oz

ⓖ part of GI symbol program   ★ little or no carbs

HOUSEHOLD MEASURE	CALORIES	FAT (g)	SATURATED FAT (g)	CARBO-HYDRATE (g)	FIBER (g)	SODIUM (mg)
1 cup	40	3	0	2	1	180
1 cup	45	3.5	0	3	1	180
1 cup	40	3	0	2	1	180
1 cup	40	3	0	2	1	180
1 cup	158	3	2	25	0	152
1 small carton	120	4	3	15	0	69
1 tbsp	82	2	2	14	0	27
1 cup	150	8	5	12	0	98
1 cup	105	3	2	12	0	127
1 cup	120	5	3	12	0	100
1 cup	134	3	0	16	0	174
1 cup	133	1	0	17	0	143
1 cup	206	9	6	24	0	98
1 std serve	52	0	0	12	0	10
1 cup	85	0	0	12	0	103
¾ cup	116	4	3	15	0	65

DAIRY PRODUCTS: MILK & ALTERNATIVES

FOOD	GI	LOW MED HIGH	SERVING SIZE
Vitasoy® Rice Milk, Original	79	high	8 fl oz
Vitasoy® Organic soy milk	43	low	8 fl oz
Vitasoy® Vita Go Banana Honey	29	low	8 fl oz
Vitasoy® Vita Go Chocolate	29	low	8 fl oz
Vitasoy® Soy Milky Chocolate	31	low	8 fl oz
Yakult®, fermented milk drink with *Lactobacillus casei*	46	low	2.2 fl oz
Yakult® Light, fermented milk drink with *Lactobacillus casei*	36	low	2.2 fl oz

@ part of GI symbol program   ★ little or no carbs

HOUSEHOLD MEASURE	CALORIES	FAT (g)	SATURATED FAT (g)	CARBO-HYDRATE (g)	FIBER (g)	SODIUM (mg)
1 cup	125	3	0	24	<1	162
1 cup	120	4	1	16	3	30
1 cup	200	5	1	29	4	50
1 cup	200	5	1	29	4	105
1 cup	140	4	1	19	<1	218
1 bottle	52	0	0	12	0	10
1 bottle	35	0	0	9	2	10

DAIRY PRODUCTS: YOGURT

FOOD	GI	LOW MED HIGH	SERVING SIZE
Yogurt, low fat, natural, plain	35	low	7 oz
Yogurt, low fat, no added sugar, vanilla or fruit	20	low	7 oz
Yoplait Original Mixed Berry yogurt	25	low	3½ oz
Yoplait Original French Vanilla yogurt	27	low	3½ oz
Yoplait Original Mango yogurt	37	low	3½ oz
Yoplait Original Strawberry yogurt	25	low	3½ oz
Yoplait Light Apple Turnover yogurt	18	low	7 oz
Yoplait Light Apricot Mango yogurt	20	low	7 oz
Yoplait Light Banana Cream Pie yogurt	18	low	7 oz
Yoplait Light Red Raspberry yogurt	16	low	7 oz
Yoplait Light Strawberry yogurt	16	low	7 oz

@ part of GI symbol program   ★ little or no carbs

HOUSEHOLD MEASURE	CALORIES	FAT (g)	SATURATED FAT (g)	CARBO-HYDRATE (g)	FIBER (g)	SODIUM (mg)
1 container	111	0	0	15	0	153
1 container	156	1	0	17	0	230
½ container	90	1	1	17	0	77
½ container	94	1	1	17	0	40
½ container	85	1	1	17	0	40
½ container	85	1	1	17	0	40
1 container	100	0	0	19	0	85
1 container	100	0	0	19	0	85
1 container	110	0	0	20	0	90
1 container	100	0	0	19	0	85
1 container	100	0	0	19	0	85

FRUIT

FOOD	GI	LOW MED HIGH	SERVING SIZE
Apple	38	low	4 oz
Apple, canned, solid pack without juice	42	low	4½ oz
Apple, dried	29	low	1 oz
Apricots	31	low	6 oz
Apricots, canned, in light syrup	64	med	4½ oz
Apricots, dried	31	low	1 oz
Apricot halves, canned in fruit juice	51	low	4½ oz
Avocado	★		2¾ oz
Banana	52	low	3 oz
Breadfruit	68	med	2 oz
Blueberries, wild	53	low	3½ oz
Cantaloupe	65	med	12 oz
Cherimoya	54	low	3 oz
Cherries, dark	63	med	4½ oz
Cherries, dried, tart	58	med	1½ oz
Cherries, frozen, tart	22	low	3½ oz
Cherries, raw, sour	22	low	5 oz
Cherries, sour, pitted, canned	41	low	4 oz
Cranberries, sweetened, dried (Ocean Spray®)	62	med	1 oz
Dates, Medjool, vacuum-packed	39	low	2 oz
Dates, pitted	39–45	low	1 oz
Figs, dried	61	med	1 oz
Fruit and nut mix	15	low	1¼ oz

@ part of GI symbol program   ★ little or no carbs

HOUSEHOLD MEASURE	CALORIES	FAT (g)	SATURATED FAT (g)	CARBO-HYDRATE (g)	FIBER (g)	SODIUM (mg)
1 small	58	0	0	13	2	1
½ cup	50	0	0	10	2	6
4 rings	69	0	0	16	2	1
2 large	70	0	0	13	4	3
½ cup	72	0	0	16	2	3
10 pieces	75	0	0	16	3	13
½ cup	58	0	0	12	1	7
⅓ average	171	18	4	0	1	2
1 small	73	0	0	16	2	1
¼ cup	57	0	0	26	3	1
½ cup	45	0	0	9	4	0
2 cups	80	0	0	16	3	34
¼ large fruit	64	1	0	13	2	3
1 cup	73	0	0	15	2	1
¼ cup	153	0	0	30	3	4
⅔ cup	50	0	0	6	1	18
1 cup	78	1	0	22	3	5
½ cup	93	0	0	21	1	5
2 tbsp	87	0	0	16	1	1
3 medium	78	0	0	18	3	4
5 average	72	0	0	17	2	4
2 medium	78	0	0	16	4	12
¼ cup	158	8	2	17	3	19

FRUIT

FOOD	GI	LOW MED HIGH	SERVING SIZE
Fruit cocktail, canned	55	low	5 oz
Fruit salad, canned in fruit juice	54	low	4½ oz
Grapefruit	25	low	11 oz
Grapefruit, ruby red segments in juice	47	low	4½ oz
Grapes	46	low	3½ oz
Kiwi	53	low	6¾ oz
Kumquats	★		¾ oz
Lemon	★		½ oz
Lime	★		½ oz
Loganberries	★		2½ oz
Lychees, canned, in syrup, drained	79	high	3 oz
Lychees, fresh, B3 variety	57	med	2 oz
Mandarin segments in juice	47	low	4½ oz
Mango	51	low	3½ oz
Mixed fruit, dried	60	med	1 oz
Mixed nuts and raisins	21	low	1 oz
Mulberries	★		2½ oz
Nectarine, fresh	43	low	4 oz
Orange	42	low	7 oz
Orange & grapefruit segments in juice	53	low	4½ oz
Papaya	59	med	5 oz
Peach	42	low	7 oz
Peach and pineapple in fruit juice	45	low	4½ oz

@ part of GI symbol program   ★ little or no carbs

HOUSEHOLD MEASURE	CALORIES	FAT (g)	SATURATED FAT (g)	CARBO-HYDRATE (g)	FIBER (g)	SODIUM (mg)
½ cup	68	0	0	16	2	5
½ cup	69	0	0	15	2	6
1 large	86	1	0	15	2	12
½ cup	77	0	0	20	1	4
25 grapes (1 small bunch)	63	0	0	15	1	6
2 small	108	0	0	19	8	11
1 average	13	0	0	2	1	1
1 wedge	2	0	0	0	0	0
1 wedge	3	0	0	0	0	0
½ cup	51	0	0	4	6	1
7 average	65	0	0	15	1	5
5 lychees	32	0	0	7	1	0
½ cup	49	0	0	12	1	7
½ average	60	0	0	13	2	1
2 tbsp	78	0	0	18	2	22
¼ cup	158	8	2	17	3	19
½ cup	23	0	0	3	2	4
1 average	50	0	0	10	2	0
1 large	78	0	0	15	4	4
½ cup	74	0	0	19	1	12
1 small	59	0	0	12	3	5
2 small	69	0	0	13	3	4
½ cup	59	0	0	13	2	6

FRUIT

FOOD	GI	LOW MED HIGH	SERVING SIZE
Peaches, canned, in heavy syrup	58	med	5 oz
Peaches, canned, in light syrup	52	med	4½ oz
Peaches, canned, in natural juice	38	low	5½ oz
Peaches, dried	35	low	1 oz
Peaches and grapes, canned in fruit juice	46	low	4½ oz
Pear	38	low	4 oz
Pear, canned, in fruit juice	44	low	4½ oz
Pear, canned, in natural juice	43	low	5 oz
Pear, dried	43	low	1 oz
Pear halves, canned, in reduced-sugar syrup, lite	25	low	3½ oz
Pineapple	59	med	6 oz
Pineapple & papaya pieces, canned in juice	53	low	4½ oz
Pineapple pieces, canned in fruit juice	43	low	4½ oz
Plum	39	low	9 oz
Prunes, pitted, Sunsweet	29	low	1½ oz
Raisins	64	med	¾ oz
Raspberries	★		2 oz
Rhubarb, stewed, unsweetened	★		3½ oz
Strawberries	40	low	17 oz
Tropical fruit and nut mix	49	low	1 oz
Watermelon	72	high	10 oz

@ part of GI symbol program   ★ little or no carbs

HOUSEHOLD MEASURE	CALORIES	FAT (g)	SATURATED FAT (g)	CARBO-HYDRATE (g)	FIBER (g)	SODIUM (mg)
½ cup	66	0	0	14	2	7
½ cup	73	0	0	17	2	4
¾ cup	69	0	0	15	2	8
3 halves	80	0	0	16	3	5
½ cup	55	0	0	13	2	5
1 small	68	0	0	16	3	2
½ cup	62	0	0	14	2	5
¾ pear	65	0	0	15	2	7
1½ halves	68	0	0	16	3	3
½ pear	62	0	0	15	2	2
1 large slice	69	2	0	13	4	3
½ cup	68	0	0	18	2	6
½ cup	74	0	0	19	2	15
2 large	103	0	0	19	6	5
5 prunes	97	0	0	22	3	38
6 tsp	60	0	0	14	1	12
½ cup	29	0	0	3	3	1
⅓ cup	19	0	0	1	3	9
3 cups	115	1	0	13	11	29
3 tbsp	120	4	1	17	1	14
1 large slice	69	1	0	14	2	6

GLUTEN-FREE PRODUCTS

FOOD	GI	LOW MED HIGH	SERVING SIZE
Apricot and Apple Fruit Strips	29	low	¾ oz
Apricot spread, no added sugar	29	low	1 oz
Buckwheat pancakes, gluten-free, packet mix	102	high	¾ oz
Cookie, chocolate-coated	35	low	1½ oz
Corn pasta	78	high	2 oz
Corn Thins, puffed corn cakes, gluten-free	87	high	¾ oz
Country Life, Low GI, gluten-free bread	40	low	1 oz
Gluten-free buckwheat bread	72	high	1 oz
Marmalade spread, no added sugar	27	low	1 oz
Muesli Breakfast Bar, gluten-free	50	low	¾ oz
Multigrain bread, gluten-free	79	high	1 oz
Pancakes, gluten-free, made from packet mix	61	med	3 oz
Pasta, rice and corn, dry	76	high	1 oz
Peach and Pear Fruit Strips	29	low	¾ oz
Plum and Apple Fruit Strips	29	low	1 oz
Raspberry spread, no added sugar	26	low	1 oz
Rice pasta, enriched (Gluten, Maize, Wheat and Soy free)	51	low	¾ oz
Spaghetti, enriched (Gluten, Wheat and Soy free)	51	low	¾ oz
Strawberry spread, no added sugar	29	low	1 oz

@ part of GI symbol program   ★ little or no carbs

HOUSEHOLD MEASURE	CALORIES	FAT (g)	SATURATED FAT (g)	CARBO-HYDRATE (g)	FIBER (g)	SODIUM (mg)
1 strip	71	0	0	16	2	5
1 tbsp	56	0	0	13	0	3
1 small	67	0	0	15	1	95
2 cookies	183	11	6	18	3	52
½ cup	78	1	0	15	3	0
4 slices	89	1	0	16	2	60
1 slice	163	6	1	20	6	183
1 slice	60	1	0	11	1	194
1 tbsp	61	0	0	14	0	3
½ bar	97	4	2	13	2	6
1 slice	91	2	1	15	2	83
2 pancakes	240	2	0	53	6	640
⅙ cup	79	0	0	19	1	2
1 strip	71	0	0	15	3	14
1½ strips	77	0	0	16	4	10
1 tbsp	60	0	0	14	0	17
⅙ cup	80	0	0	18	1	3
⅙ cup	79	0	0	19	1	3
1 tbsp	60	0	0	14	0	3

MEALS, PREPARED & CONVENIENCE

FOOD	GI	LOW MED HIGH	SERVING SIZE
Baked potato with baked beans	62	med	7 oz
Beef and ale casserole, prepared convenience meal	53	low	10½ oz
Burrito, made with corn tortilla, refried beans and tomato salsa	39	low	3½ oz
Cannelloni, spinach and ricotta, prepared convenience meal	15	low	8 oz
Chicken curry and rice, prepared convenience meal	45	low	10½ oz
Chicken fajitas	42	low	3 oz
Chicken nuggets, frozen, reheated in microwave 5 mins	46	low	4 oz
Chicken tandoori curry with rice, prepared meal	45	low	10 oz
Chow mein, chicken, prepared convenience meal	51	low	10½ oz
Creamy carbonara whole grain pasta & sauce meal	39	low	5 oz
Fish fingers	38	low	2½ oz
French fries, frozen, reheated in microwave	75	high	5 oz
French-style chicken with rice, prepared convenience meal	36	low	7 oz
Grape leaves, stuffed with rice and lamb, served with tomato sauce	30	low	4 oz

© part of GI symbol program ★ little or no carbs

HOUSEHOLD MEASURE	CALORIES	FAT (g)	SATURATED FAT (g)	CARBO-HYDRATE (g)	FIBER (g)	SODIUM (mg)
1 medium potato	147	1	0	26	6	251
1 meal	444	23	10	17	3	657
1 small burrito	264	13	6	19	2	688
1 serving	196	4	2	30	4	573
1 meal	640	48	26	20	3	198
1 fajita	138	8	3.8	6	2	175
6 nuggets	288	17	7	16	1	454
1 meal	488	22	12	53	2	455
1 meal	448	33	12	18	8	990
1 serving	148	5	2	21	2	290
3 fingers	156	8	2	13	1	220
10 fries	120	3	0	19	2	25
1 serving	287	11	3	32	2	394
4 stuffed leaves	124	4	2	15	2	268

MEALS, PREPARED & CONVENIENCE

FOOD	GI	LOW MED HIGH	SERVING SIZE
Hamburger, commercially prepared	66	med	3 oz
Lamb moussaka, prepared convenience meal	35	low	10½ oz
Lasagna, beef, commercially made	47	low	5 oz
Mashed potato, instant	85	high	4 oz
McDonald's Chicken McNuggets® consumed with Sweet 'N Sour Sauce	55	low	4½ oz
McDonald's Filet-O-Fish®	66	med	4½ oz
McDonald's Hamburger	66	med	3½ oz
McDonald's McChicken®	66	med	6½ oz
Pizza, cheese	60	med	5 oz
Pizza, Super Supreme, pan, Pizza Hut	36	low	1¾ oz
Pizza, Super Supreme, Thin 'n Crispy, Pizza Hut	30	low	2½ oz
Pizza, Veggie Lovers®, Thin 'n Crispy, Pizza Hut	49	low	1¾ oz
President's Choice® Blue Menu™ Cauliflower Topped Shepherd's Pie	21	low	8 oz
President's Choice® Blue Menu™ Pasta Sauce, Tomato and Basil	33	low	4 oz
President's Choice® Blue Menu™ Penne with Roasted Vegetable Entrée	39	low	11 oz

@ part of GI symbol program   ★ little or no carbs

HOUSEHOLD MEASURE	CALORIES	FAT (g)	SATURATED FAT (g)	CARBO-HYDRATE (g)	FIBER (g)	SODIUM (mg)
1 small burger	254	10	3	28	1	378
1 meal	312	19	4	20	6	620
1 serving	190	8	4	17	4	330
½ cup	74	0	0	14	2	4
6 nuggets & sauce	333	18	3	26	1	627
1 sandwich	310	14	3	30	2	634
1 small burger	237	9	4	25	2	433
1 sandwich	418	19	3	40	2	706
2 slices	429	18	6	52	3	266
1/16 of large pizza	127	5	2	14	1	241
1/8 of large pizza	197	8	4	18	2	566
1/16 of large pizza	123	4	2	15	1	284
¼ pie	220	9	5	13	1	590
½ cup	70	2	0	8	2	480
1 container	320	6	3	43	9	750

MEALS, PREPARED & CONVENIENCE

FOOD	GI	LOW MED HIGH	SERVING SIZE
President's Choice® Blue Menu™ Vegetarian Chili	39	low	8 oz
Sausages	28	low	4 oz
Sausages and mashed potato, prepared convenience meal	61	med	10 oz
Shepherd's pie	66	med	10½ oz
Sirloin steak with mixed vegetables and mashed potato, homemade	66	med	10½ oz
Spaghetti bolognese, homemade	52	low	10½ oz
Spring Roll, vegetable, baked	50	low	3 oz
Stir-fried vegetables with chicken and boiled white rice, homemade	73	high	10½ oz
Sushi, salmon	48	low	2¾ oz
Taco shells, cornmeal-based, baked	68	med	1 oz
Tofu and pickled radish nori roll with brown rice	45	low	7 oz

@ part of GI symbol program   ★ little or no carbs

HOUSEHOLD MEASURE	CALORIES	FAT (g)	SATURATED FAT (g)	CARBO-HYDRATE (g)	FIBER (g)	SODIUM (mg)
1 cup	200	3	1	34	5	480
2 sausages	303	21	10	9	3	1079
1 meal	256	13	6	27	6	1305
1 meal	320	16	7	22	3	1275
1 meal	309	13	5	25	6	122
1 meal	468	11	4	65	5	420
1 roll	96	2	0	18	3	321
1 meal	344	4	1	62	5	319
3 pieces	102	1	0	19	1	291
2 regular size	120	6	1	16	2	95
1 roll	215	3	0	42	2	162

MEAT, SEAFOOD, EGGS & PROTEIN

FOOD	GI	LOW MED HIGH	SERVING SIZE
Bacon, fried	★		1 oz
Bacon, grilled	★		1 oz
Beef, corned silverside	★		¾ oz
Beef, corned silverside, canned	★		1¾ oz
Beef, roast	★		1 oz
Beef steak, fat trimmed	★		6 oz
Burger, fried	★		1¾ oz
Calamari, fried	★		2 oz
Calamari rings, squid, not battered or crumbed	★		3 oz
Chicken breast, baked without skin	★		3 oz
Chicken breast, grilled without skin	★		3 oz
Chicken chopped, cooked	★		3½ oz
Chicken drumstick, grilled without skin	★		1½ oz
Chicken loaf	★		¾ oz
Chicken roll	★		¾ oz
Chicken thigh fillet grilled, without skin	★		1¾ oz
Chicken wing grilled, without skin	★		¾ oz
Cod, fried	★		4 oz
Crab, cooked	★		2 oz
Duck, roasted, without skin	★		2 oz

@ part of GI symbol program   ★ little or no carbs

HOUSEHOLD MEASURE	CALORIES	FAT (g)	SATURATED FAT (g)	CARBOHYDRATE (g)	FIBER (g)	SODIUM (mg)
1 small slice	38	2	1	1	0	500
1 slice	49	2	1	1	0	735
1 slice	23	1	1	0	0	213
2 slices	96	6	2	0	0	570
2 slices	44	1	1	0	0	17
1 medium	356	17	7	0	0	119
1 average	101	6	1	3	0	241
½ cup	70	3	1	0	0	192
5 rings	78	1	0	2	0	37
⅓ small	140	6	2	0	0	65
⅓ small	150	7	2	0	0	70
½ cup	204	11	3	0	0	101
1 small	78	3	1	0	0	50
1 slice	42	2	1	2	0	172
1 slice	31	2	1	1	0	142
½ large	113	7	2	0	0	55
1 medium	37	2	1	0	0	19
1 fillet	192	10	3	3	1	163
½ cup	68	0	0	1	0	218
½ breast	156	8	2	0	0	81

MEAT, SEAFOOD, EGGS & PROTEIN

FOOD	GI	LOW MED HIGH	SERVING SIZE
Egg, whole, raw	★		2 fl oz
Egg white, raw	★		1 fl oz
Egg yolk, raw	★		½ fl oz
Flounder, fried	★		4 oz
Frankfurter	★		2 oz
Ham, canned leg	★		1½ oz
Hamburger patty	★		2¾ oz
Kingfish (Mackerel), fried	★		4 oz
Lamb, ground, cooked	★		3½ oz
Lamb, grilled chop, fat trimmed	★		1¾ oz
Lamb, roasted loin, fat trimmed	★		2 oz
Ling (Lingcod), fried	★		4 oz
Liver, cooked	★		2 oz
Liverwurst	★		1 oz
Lobster, cooked	★		2 oz
Mullet, fried	★		4 oz
Mussels, cooked	★		2 oz
Nutolene	★		3 oz
Ocean perch, fried	★		4 oz
Octopus, cooked	★		2 oz
Oysters, natural, plain	★		3 oz
Pancetta	★		¾ oz
Pepperoni	★		¾ oz
Pork, grilled chops, fat trimmed	★		3 oz

@ part of GI symbol program   ★ little or no carbs

HOUSEHOLD MEASURE	CALORIES	FAT (g)	SATURATED FAT (g)	CARBO-HYDRATE (g)	FIBER (g)	SODIUM (mg)
1 average	77	6	2	0	0	72
1 average	15	0	0	0	0	54
1 average	53	5	2	0	0	10
1 fillet	201	10	3	3	1	148
1 average	144	11	4	1	0	439
1 thick slice	45	2	1	0	0	500
1 patty	197	14	6	0	0	52
1 fillet	261	13	4	4	1	136
½ cup	218	13	7	0	0	80
1 medium	108	5	3	0	0	36
1 thick slice	141	10	5	0	0	34
1 fillet	204	10	3	3	1	230
½ cup	158	8	3	2	0	53
2 slices	92	8	3	0	0	244
½ cup	53	1	0	0	0	213
1 fillet	281	17	6	4	1	234
½ cup	76	2	1	4	1	562
2 thick slices	214	18	3	4	2	281
1 fillet	210	10	3	4	1	147
½ cup	69	1	0	1	0	204
6 medium	57	2	1	3	0	177
1 slice	40	3	1	0	0	275
1 slice	106	9	4	1	0	365
1 medium	171	7	3	0	0	71

MEAT, SEAFOOD, EGGS & PROTEIN

FOOD	GI	LOW MED HIGH	SERVING SIZE
Prosciutto	★		1½ oz
Quail	★		2¾ oz
Salami	★		¾ oz
Salmon, pink, no added salt, drained	★		2 oz
Salmon, red, no added salt, drained	★		2 oz
Sardines, canned in oil, drained	★		2 oz
Sausages, fried	★		2 oz
Scallops, cooked	★		2 oz
Seafood marinara, canned	★		2 oz
Shark, fried	★		4 oz
Shrimp	★		1 oz
Shrimp, cooked	★		2 oz
Snapper, fried	★		4 oz
Sole, fried	★		4 oz
Spam, lite	★		2 oz
Spam, regular	★		1½ oz
Speck	★		3½ oz
Steak, lean	★		7 oz
Tofu, plain, unsweetened	★		3½ oz
Tofu, cooked	★		4½ oz
Trout, cooked	★		4 oz
Trout, fresh or frozen	★		5¾ oz

@ part of GI symbol program   ★ little or no carbs

HOUSEHOLD MEASURE	CALORIES	FAT (g)	SATURATED FAT (g)	CARBO-HYDRATE (g)	FIBER (g)	SODIUM (mg)
1 slice	51	2	1	0	0	753
1 average	151	7	2	0	0	45
1 slice	98	9	3	0	0	336
⅔ small can	90	4	1	0	0	67
⅔ small can	119	7	2	0	0	67
⅔ small can	137	10	3	0	0	372
1 sausage	239	17	8	4	2	928
½ cup	56	1	0	0	0	91
⅔ small can	67	1	0	3	1	367
1 fillet	231	9	2	3	1	164
4 large shrimp	28	0	0	0	0	63
½ cup	55	1	0	0	0	228
1 fillet	251	12	4	4	1	181
1 fillet	206	11	3	3	1	186
2 slices	96	8	3	2	0	580
2 slices	133	12	5	1	0	628
1 slice	212	14	5	0	0	1480
1 medium steak	238	10	5	0	0	72
1 serve	127	7	1	0	7	40
½ cup	96	6	1	1	0	5
1 fillet	164	6	1	0	0	70
1 medium trout	238	8	2	0	0	104

MEAT, SEAFOOD, EGGS & PROTEIN

FOOD	GI	LOW MED HIGH	SERVING SIZE
Trout, fried	★		4 oz
Tuna, cooked	★		4 oz
Tuna in brine, drained	★		2 oz
Tuna in oil	★		2 oz
Turkey breast, deli-sliced	★		¾ oz
Turkey breast, rolled roast	★		3 oz
Turkey breast, smoked, without skin	★		3 oz
Turkey leg, roasted without skin	★		3 oz
Turkey, roasted breast without skin	★		2¾ oz
Veal, roasted, fat trimmed	★		3 oz
Vegetarian sausages	★		3 oz

@ part of GI symbol program   ★ little or no carbs

HOUSEHOLD MEASURE	CALORIES	FAT (g)	SATURATED FAT (g)	CARBO-HYDRATE (g)	FIBER (g)	SODIUM (mg)
1 fillet	200	9	3	4	1	129
1 fillet	213	8	3	0	0	57
⅔ small can	76	2	1	0	0	253
⅔ small can	177	14	2	0	0	253
1 slice	34	1	0	0	0	46
2 thick slices	132	3	1	0	0	179
2 thick slices	132	3	1	0	0	179
2 thick slices	146	6	2	0	0	145
2 thick slices	117	3	1	0	0	158
2 thick slices	122	1	0	0	0	43
1 thick	109	4	1	3	2	381

NUTRITIONAL SUPPLEMENTS

FOOD	GI	LOW MED HIGH	SERVING SIZE
Ensure Plus™, vanilla	40	low	8 fl oz
Ensure®, vanilla drink	48	low	8 fl oz
Jevity® 1 cal, unflavored	48	low	8 fl oz
Jevity® 1.2 cal, unflavored	59	med	8 fl oz
Promote with Fiber™ nutritional supplement	49	low	8 fl oz
ProSure™, ready-to-drink nutritional supplement, vanilla flavor	55	low	8 fl oz
TwoCal HN™, high nitrogen nutritional supplement, vanilla flavor	55	low	8 fl oz

@ part of GI symbol program   ★ little or no carbs

HOUSEHOLD MEASURE	CALORIES	FAT (g)	SATURATED FAT (g)	CARBO-HYDRATE (g)	FIBER (g)	SODIUM (mg)
1 bottle	350	11	1	47	3	220
1 bottle	250	6	1	40	0	200
1 can	250	8	2	33	1	220
1 can	285	9	2	36	4	325
1 can	237	7	2	30	3	310
1 can	300	7	2	41	3	360
1 can	475	22	5	51	1	345

NUTS & SEEDS

FOOD	GI	LOW MED HIGH	SERVING SIZE
Almonds, raw	24	low	½ oz
Almonds, roasted	24	low	½ oz
Blue Diamond Whole Natural Almonds	25	low	1 oz
Brazil nuts	24		½ oz
Cashew nuts, raw	22	low	½ oz
Cashew nuts, roasted and salted	22	low	½ oz
Coconut, fresh	★		½ oz
Coconut cream	★		4 fl oz
Coconut milk, canned	★		4 fl oz
Coconut milk, fresh	★		4 fl oz
Flaxseeds	32	low	½ oz
Hazelnuts	24	low	½ oz
Macadamia nuts, raw	24	low	½ oz
Macadamia nuts, roasted	24	low	½ oz
Mixed nuts, fruit, seeds	21	low	½ oz
Mixed nuts, raw	24	low	½ oz
Mixed nuts, roasted, salted	24	low	½ oz
Mixed nuts, roasted, unsalted	24	low	½ oz
Nut & raisin mix	15	low	½ oz
Nut & seed mix	★		½ oz
Peanut butter	14	low	½ oz
Peanut butter, no added sugar	14	low	½ oz
Peanuts, raw	23	low	1 oz

@ part of GI symbol program   ★ little or no carbs

HOUSEHOLD MEASURE	CALORIES	FAT (g)	SATURATED FAT (g)	CARBO-HYDRATE (g)	FIBER (g)	SODIUM (mg)
1 tbsp	79	7	1	1	1	1
1 tbsp	84	8	1	1	1	1
24 nuts	160	14	1	6	3	0
1 tbsp	90	9	2	0	1	0
1 tbsp	76	6	1	2	1	1
1 tbsp	83	7	1	3	1	38
1 tbsp	37	4	3	1	1	2
½ cup	263	26	23	5	2	27
½ cup	261	26	23	5	2	27
½ cup	302	30	27	4	3	19
1 tbsp	46	3	0	2	3	7
1 tbsp	84	8	0	1	1	0
1 tbsp	96	10	1	1	1	0
1 tbsp	96	10	1	1	1	72
1 tbsp	62	4	1	4	1	5
1 tbsp	79	7	1	1	1	0
1 tbsp	84	7	1	4	1	95
1 tbsp	81	7	1	4	1	0
1 tbsp	68	5	1	5	1	21
1 tbsp	81	7	1	1	1	21
3 tsp	104	8	1	2	1	51
3 tsp	107	9	2	1	2	51
1 tbsp	155	13	2	3	2	0

NUTS & SEEDS

FOOD	GI	LOW MED HIGH	SERVING SIZE
Peanuts, roasted	23	low	½ oz
Pecans, raw	24	low	½ oz
Pine nuts	24	low	½ oz
Pistachio nuts, raw	24	low	½ oz
Pistachio nuts, roasted	24	low	½ oz
Poppy seeds	★		¼ oz
Pumpkin seeds, raw	10	low	½ oz
Sesame seeds	18	low	⅓ oz
Sunflower seeds, raw	★		½ oz
Sunflower seeds, roasted	★		½ oz
Walnuts	★		½ oz

ⓖ part of GI symbol program   ★ little or no carbs

HOUSEHOLD MEASURE	CALORIES	FAT (g)	SATURATED FAT (g)	CARBO-HYDRATE (g)	FIBER (g)	SODIUM (mg)
1 tbsp	115	10	1	3	1	61
1 tbsp	93	9	1	2	1	0
1 tbsp	91	9	1	1	1	0
1 tbsp	79	7	1	2	1	1
1 tbsp	77	6	1	2	1	83
2 tsp	26	2	0	0	1	1
1 tbsp	75	6	1	2	1	2
1 tbsp	52	4	1	1	1	1
1 tbsp	75	7	1	0	1	0
1 tbsp	77	7	1	0	1	81
1 tbsp	90	9	1	0	1	0

OILS & DRESSINGS

FOOD	GI	LOW MED HIGH	SERVING SIZE
Caesar salad dressing	★		1 fl oz
Canola oil	★		⅓ fl oz
Cream, pure, >35% fat	★		1 fl oz
Cream, sour, >35% fat	★		1 oz
Cream, thickened, >35% fat	★		¾ fl oz
Dripping, pork	★		⅓ fl oz
French dressing	★		1 fl oz
French dressing, fat free, artificially sweetened	★		1 fl oz
Ghee	★		⅓ oz
Italian dressing	★		1 fl oz
Italian dressing, fat free, artificially sweetened	★		1 fl oz
Lard	★		⅓ oz
Margarine, cooking	★		⅓ oz
Mayonnaise	★		½ fl oz
Mayonnaise, creamy, 97% fat free	★		¾ fl oz
Salad dressing, homemade oil & vinegar	★		1 fl oz
Safflower oil	★		⅓ fl oz
Sesame oil	★		⅓ fl oz
Soybean oil	★		⅓ fl oz
Sunflower oil	★		⅓ fl oz
Tartar sauce	★		1 fl oz
Thousand Island dressing	★		¾ fl oz
Vinegar	★		½ fl oz

@ part of GI symbol program   ★ little or no carbs

HOUSEHOLD MEASURE	CALORIES	FAT (g)	SATURATED FAT (g)	CARBO-HYDRATE (g)	FIBER (g)	SODIUM (mg)
1½ tbsp	149	17	2	0	0	6
2 tsp	89	10	1	0	0	0
1½ tbsp	120	13	9	1	0	6
1½ tbsp	120	13	8	1	0	9
1 tbsp	70	7	5	1	0	10
2 tsp	83	9	4	0	0	0
1½ tbsp	82	7	1	4	0	567
1½ tbsp	3	0	0	0	0	514
2 tsp	97	11	7	0	0	0
1½ tbsp	95	9	1	2	0	399
1½ tbsp	4	0	0	0	0	239
2 tsp	83	9	4	0	0	0
2 tsp	72	8	4	0	0	113
1 tbsp	56	5	1	3	0	122
1 tbsp	24	1	0	5	0	152
1½ tbsp	178	20	2	0	0	7
2 tsp	89	10	1	0	0	0
2 tsp	89	10	1	0	0	0
2 tsp	89	10	2	0	0	0
2 tsp	89	10	1	0	0	0
1½ tbsp	71	7	1	2	0	157
1 tbsp	56	5	1	4	0	210
1 tbsp	3	0	0	0	0	1

PASTA & NOODLES

FOOD	GI	LOW MED HIGH	SERVING SIZE
Beef ravioli, fresh, commercially made	43	low	5 oz
Beef & vegetable ravioli, fresh, commercially made	47	low	5 oz
Meat pasta sauce	24	low	6 oz
Cannelloni, spinach and ricotta, prepared convenience meal	15	low	8 oz
Capellini pasta, white, boiled	45	low	2 oz
Cheese & vegetable ravioli, fresh, commercially made	51	low	5 oz
Cheese tortellini, cooked	50	low	1¾ oz
Chicken & garlic ravioli, fresh, commercially made	44	low	5 oz
Corn pasta, gluten-free, boiled	78	high	1¾ oz
Couscous, boiled 5 mins	65	med	5½ oz
Creamy carbonara whole-grain pasta & sauce meal	39	low	5 oz
Creamy sun-dried tomato pasta sauce	19	low	6 oz
Fettuccine, egg, fresh	40	low	5 oz
Fusilli twists, tricolor, boiled	51	low	2½ oz
Gnocchi, cooked	68	med	1¾ oz
@ Israeli Couscous, Osem brand, boiled	52	low	2.2 oz
Italian tomato & garlic pasta sauce	40	low	6 oz
Lasagna, beef, commercially made	47	low	5 oz
Lasagna sheets, fresh	49	low	2½ oz

@ part of GI symbol program   ★ little or no carbs

HOUSEHOLD MEASURE	CALORIES	FAT (g)	SATURATED FAT (g)	CARBO-HYDRATE (g)	FIBER (g)	SODIUM (mg)
1 serving	279	8	4	40	3	620
1 serving	330	9	4	45	5	550
1 serving	154	6	2	13	0	743
1 serving	196	4	2	30	4	573
⅓ cup	74	0	0	15	1	34
1 serving	300	5	2	46	4	649
⅓ cup	98	2	0	15	1	115
1 serving	263	6	2	38	3	508
⅓ cup	59	0	0	13	2	0
1 cup	73	0	0	15	0	2
1 serving	148	5	2	21	2	290
1 serving	178	12	8	15	0	354
1 cup	204	3	1	36	3	4
½ cup	90	0	0	19	1	35
¼ cup	74	1	0	15	1	30
½ cup	94	0	0	20	1	1
1 serving	127	8	1	12	0	513
1 serving	190	8	4	17	4	330
2 sheets	137	3	1	22	6	4

PASTA & NOODLES

FOOD	GI	LOW MED HIGH	SERVING SIZE
Linguine, thick, durum wheat, boiled	46	low	2 oz
Linguine, thin, durum wheat, boiled	52	low	2 oz
Macaroni, white, durum wheat, boiled	47	low	2 oz
Macaroni and cheese, from packet mix, Kraft	64	med	2½ oz
Mediterranean pasta sauce	40	low	6 oz
More Than Pasta Fettuccine Pasta (fresh pasta)	31	low	2 oz
Mung bean noodles, dried, boiled	33	low	1¾ oz
Noodles, dried rice, boiled	61	med	2½ oz
Noodles, fresh rice, boiled	40	low	2½ oz
President's Choice® Blue Menu™ 100% Whole Wheat Lasagna pasta	46	low	3 oz
President's Choice® Blue Menu™ 100% Whole Wheat Penne Rigate pasta	51	low	3¼ oz
President's Choice® Blue Menu™ 100% Whole Wheat Spaghetti pasta	45	low	3¼ oz
President's Choice® Blue Menu™ 100% Whole Wheat Spaghettini	56	med	3¼ oz
President's Choice® Blue Menu™ Fettuccini	55	low	4 oz

@ part of GI symbol program   ★ little or no carbs

HOUSEHOLD MEASURE	CALORIES	FAT (g)	SATURATED FAT (g)	CARBO-HYDRATE (g)	FIBER (g)	SODIUM (mg)
⅓ cup	74	0	0	15	1	34
⅓ cup	74	0	0	15	1	34
⅓ cup	74	0	0	15	1	34
⅛ packet	138	5	4	19	1	186
1 serving	130	7	1	8	0	602
¼ package	150	1	0	22	5	180
⅓ cup	53	0	0	13	1	2
⅓ cup	75	0	0	16	0	11
⅓ cup	81	0	0	17	0	11
4 sheets	310	2	0	56	7	2
⅕ package	330	2	1	56	9	2
⅕ package	330	2	1	56	9	85
⅕ package	330	2	1	56	9	2
⅓ package	340	4	1	56	6	25

PASTA & NOODLES

FOOD	GI	LOW MED HIGH	SERVING SIZE
President's Choice® Blue Menu™ Whole Grain Lasagna Sheets	52	low	2¼ oz
President's Choice® 100% Whole Wheat Rotini	57	med	3 oz
Ravioli, meat-filled, durum wheat flour, boiled	39	low	2 oz
Rice and corn pasta, gluten-free	76	high	2½ oz
Rice pasta, brown, boiled	92	high	5 oz
Rice vermicelli noodles, dried, boiled, Chinese	58	med	2 oz
Ricotta & spinach agnolotti, fresh, commercially made	47	low	5 oz
Soba noodles / buckwheat noodles	59	med	4 oz
Soba noodles, instant, served in soup	46	low	1¾ oz
Spaghetti with meat sauce, homemade	52	low	5 oz
Spaghetti, gluten-free, canned in tomato sauce	68	med	4 oz
Spaghetti, protein-enriched, boiled	27	low	1¾ oz
Spaghetti, white, durum wheat, boiled 10–15 mins	44	low	2 oz
Spaghetti, whole wheat, boiled	42	low	2 oz
Spicy tomato & bacon pasta sauce	24	low	6 oz
Spirali, white, durum wheat, boiled	43	low	2 oz
Toasted pasta, Osem brand, boiled	52	low	2.2 oz

ⓖ part of GI symbol program   ★ little or no carbs

HOUSEHOLD MEASURE	CALORIES	FAT (g)	SATURATED FAT (g)	CARBO-HYDRATE (g)	FIBER (g)	SODIUM (mg)
1½ sheets	200	3	1	34	4	35
⅓ pack	330	2	1	56	9	85
⅓ cup	114	4	2	13	3	228
⅓ cup	99	0	0	16	0	46
1 cup	210	2	1	41	3	5
⅓ cup	75	0	0	16	0	4
1 serving	279	8	5	41	3	494
1 cup	113	0	0	24	2	68
⅓ cup	62	0	0	14	1	5
1 serving	197	6	2	23	4	360
½ can	69	0	0	14	1	440
⅓ cup	77	0	0	15	1	2
⅓ cup	74	0	0	15	1	34
⅓ cup	74	0	0	15	1	34
1 serving	121	5	1	13	0	708
⅓ cup	74	0	0	15	1	34
½ cup	94	0	0	20	1	1

PASTA & NOODLES

FOOD	GI	LOW MED HIGH	SERVING SIZE
Udon noodles, plain, boiled	62	med	2 oz
Veal tortellini, fresh, commercially made	48	low	5 oz
Vermicelli pasta, white, durum wheat, boiled	35	low	2 oz
Whole grain ricotta & spinach ravioli, fresh, commercially made	39	low	5 oz

© part of GI symbol program   ★ little or no carbs

HOUSEHOLD MEASURE	CALORIES	FAT (g)	SATURATED FAT (g)	CARBO-HYDRATE (g)	FIBER (g)	SODIUM (mg)
⅓ cup	66	1	0	13	0	95
1 serving	246	6	2	37	3	437
⅓ cup	74	0	0	15	1	34
1 serving	276	8	5	37	6	734

RICE

FOOD	GI	LOW MED HIGH	SERVING SIZE
Arborio risotto rice, white, boiled, SunRice®	69	med	6.5 oz
Basmati rice, white, boiled	58	med	5.5 oz
Broken rice, Thai, white, cooked in rice cooker	86	high	6.5 oz
Brown Pelde rice, boiled	76	high	6.75 oz
Calrose rice, brown, medium-grain, boiled	87	high	6.75 oz
Calrose rice, white, medium-grain, boiled	83	high	6.5 oz
Doongara Clever rice, SunRice®	54	low	5.5 oz
Glutinous rice, white, cooked in rice cooker	98	high	6 oz
Instant rice, white, cooked 6 mins with water	87	high	6 oz
Jasmine fragrant rice, SunRice®	89	high	6 oz
Jasmine rice, white, long-grain, cooked in rice cooker	109	high	6 oz
Long-grain rice, white, Mahatma®, boiled 15 mins	50	low	5.5 oz
Moolgiri rice	54	low	5.5 oz
Pelde parboiled rice, Sungold	87	high	6 oz
Seeds of Change® Rishikesh Whole Grain Brown Basmati Rice	51	low	5 oz
Sunbrown Quick® rice, Ricegrowers, boiled	80	high	6.5 oz

HOUSEHOLD MEASURE	CALORIES	FAT (g)	SATURATED FAT (g)	CARBO-HYDRATE (g)	FIBER (g)	SODIUM (mg)
I cup	242	0	0	53	1	50
I cup	205	0	0	45	1	50
I cup	242	0	0	52	1	40
I cup	218	2	0	46	4	35
I cup	218	2	0	46	4	33
I cup	242	0	0	53	1	33
I cup	205	0	0	45	1	45
I cup	169	0	0	37	2	45
I cup	199	1	0	43	1	45
I cup	213	0	0	48	1	48
I cup	213	0	0	48	1	48
I cup	205	0	0	45	1	45
I cup	205	0	0	45	1	45
I cup	219	0	0	48	1	43
I cup	220	4	1	43	2	10
I cup	275	2	0	57	3	38

RICE

FOOD	GI	LOW MED HIGH	SERVING SIZE
SunRice®, Basmati, white rice, 2½ minute, microwave pouch	52	low	4 oz
SunRice® Japanese-Style Sushi Rice, white	85	high	6 oz
SunRice® Koshihikari rice, Ricegrowers	73	high	6 oz
SunRice®, Low GI, white, dry, boiled	54	low	2½ oz
SunRice® Medium Grain brown rice	59	med	6.75 oz
SunRice® Medium Grain Brown Rice in 90 Seconds, microwaved	59	med	4½ oz
SunRice® Medium Grain white rice, boiled	75	high	6 oz
SunRice® Long Grain White Rice in 90 Seconds, microwaved	76	high	4½ oz
SunRice® Premium White Long Grain rice	59	med	5.5 oz
Uncle Ben's® Converted® Brand Original Enriched Parboiled Long Grain Rice	55	low	5 oz
Uncle Ben's® Ready Rice® Pouch Whole Grain Brown	49	low	5 oz
Uncle Ben's® Ready Rice® Pouch Chicken Flavored Whole Grain Brown	46	low	5¼ oz
Uncle Ben's® Ready Rice® Pouch Long Grain & Wild with 23 Herbs & Seasonings	52	low	5 oz

@ part of GI symbol program ★ little or no carbs

HOUSEHOLD MEASURE	CALORIES	FAT (g)	SATURATED FAT (g)	CARBO-HYDRATE (g)	FIBER (g)	SODIUM (mg)
½ cup	169	2	0	33	2	49
1 cup	197	0	0	47	1	30
1 cup	213	0	0	48	1	48
⅓ cup	246	0	0	55	0	4
1 cup	218	2	0	46	4	33
½ cup	236	4	1	43	4	2
1 cup	221	0	0	49	1	45
½ cup	251	4	1	49	1	2
1 cup	205	0	0	45	1	45
1 cup	170	0	0	37	0	0
1 cup	240	3	0	39	2	15
1 cup	220	4	1	41	3	710
1 cup	220	3	0	43	2	900

RICE

FOOD	GI	LOW MED HIGH	SERVING SIZE
Uncle Ben's® Ready Rice® Pouch Original Enriched Long Grain White Rice	48	low	5 oz
Uncle Ben's® Ready Rice® Pouch Roasted Chicken Flavored with Carrots & Herbs	51	low	5 oz
Uncle Ben's® Ready Rice® Pouch Spanish Style with Tomatoes & Peppers	51	low	5 oz
Uncle Ben's® Ready Rice® Pouch Teriyaki Style with Peas & Carrots	45	low	5 oz
Uncle Ben's® Ready Rice® Pouch Butter & Garlic Flavored	44	low	5 oz
Uncle Ben's® Ready Whole Grain Medley™ Brown & Wild	45	low	5 oz
Uncle Ben's® Ready Whole Grain Medley™ Pouch Santa Fe Brown Rice	48	low	5 oz
Uncle Ben's® Ready Whole Grain Medley™ Pouch Vegetable Harvest	48	low	5 oz
Uncle Ben's® Ready Whole Grain Medley™ Roasted Garlic Flavored	47	low	5 oz
Uncle Ben's® Whole Grain White Rice Taco Flavor	52	low	5 oz

@ part of GI symbol program   ★ little or no carbs

HOUSEHOLD MEASURE	CALORIES	FAT (g)	SATURATED FAT (g)	CARBO-HYDRATE (g)	FIBER (g)	SODIUM (mg)
1 cup	200	3	0	40	1	10
1 cup	220	4	0	41	2	1020
1 cup	200	3	0	41	3	680
1 cup	220	3	0	42	3	870
1 cup	220	4	1	41	2	750
1 cup	220	4	0	42	3	730
1 cup	220	3	0	42	5	700
1 cup	220	3	0	44	5	780
1 cup	220	3	0	38	3	560
1 cup	160	1.5	0	35	4	570

SNACK FOODS

FOOD	GI	LOW MED HIGH	SERVING SIZE
Apricot-filled fruit bar, whole wheat pastry	50	low	1 oz
Balance Bar Gold Caramel Nut Blast	17	low	1½ oz
Balance Bar Gold Chocolate Peanut Butter	17	low	1½ oz
Balance Bar Original Chocolate Craze	17	low	1½ oz
Balance Bar Original Cookie Dough	22	low	1½ oz
Balance Bar Original Peanut Butter	25	low	1½ oz
Balance Bar Original Yogurt Honey Peanut	24	low	1½ oz
Beanitos Black Bean Chipotle BBQ Chips	42	low	1 oz
Beanitos Black Bean Chips	33	low	1 oz
Beanitos Hot Chili Lime Puffs	55	low	1 oz
Beanitos Pinto Bean & Flax Chips	44	low	1 oz
Beanitos Nacho Cheese White Bean Chips	37	low	1 oz
Beanitos Restaurant Style White Bean Chips	37	low	1 oz
Beanitos White Cheddar Puffs	48	low	1 oz
Cadbury's® milk chocolate, plain	49	low	1 oz
Cashew nuts, salted	22	low	1¾ oz
Chickpea chips	44	low	2 oz

@ part of GI symbol program   ★ little or no carbs

HOUSEHOLD MEASURE	CALORIES	FAT (g)	SATURATED FAT (g)	CARBO-HYDRATE (g)	FIBER (g)	SODIUM (mg)
1 bar	105	5	4	12	6	25
1 bar	200	7	4	22	2	160
1 bar	200	7	3.5	21	1	150
1 bar	200	7	4	21	2	160
1 bar	210	7	4	22	1	200
1 bar	200	7	3	21	1	170
1 bar	200	7	3.5	22	1	120
10 chips	140	7	0.5	15	5	150
10 chips	140	7	0.5	15	5	55
1 oz	120	4	0.5	19	4	130
10 chips	140	8	0.5	15	5	55
12 chips	140	7	1	16	6	140
12 chips	140	7	0.5	16	6	55
1 oz	120	4	0.5	18	4	180
1 row	147	8	5	16	1	36
⅓ cup	319	26	4	13	2	145
1 small packet	245	12	3	25	6	22

SNACK FOODS

FOOD	GI	LOW MED HIGH	SERVING SIZE
Chocolate brownies	42	low	2 oz
Chocolate, dark, Dove®	23	low	1 oz
Chocolate, dark, plain, regular	41	low	1 oz
Chocolate, milk, plain, Nestlé®	42	low	1 oz
Chocolate, milk, plain, reduced sugar	35	low	1 oz
Chocolate, milk, plain, regular	41	low	1 oz
Chocolate, milk, plain, with fructose instead of regular sugar	20	low	1 oz
Chocolate Raspberry Zing™ bar, Revival Soy®	47	low	1 bar
Combos® Snacks Cheddar Cheese Crackers	54	low	1¾ oz
Combos® Snacks Cheddar Cheese Pretzels	52	low	1¾ oz
Corn chips	74	high	1 oz
Corn chips, plain, salted	42	low	1 oz
Dove® milk chocolate	45	low	1 oz
Fruit and nut mix	32	low	2 oz
Granola Gourmet™ 4Real™ Energy Bar, Cran-Orange	19	low	35 g
Granola Gourmet™ 4Real™ Energy Bar, Fudge Brownie	23	low	35 g

@ part of GI symbol program   ★ little or no carbs

HOUSEHOLD MEASURE	CALORIES	FAT (g)	SATURATED FAT (g)	CARBO-HYDRATE (g)	FIBER (g)	SODIUM (mg)
1 large brownie	227	9	2	36	1	175
⅓ bar	170	11	5	23	3	0
1 row family-sized block	155	9	6	15	2	0
1 row	145	8	5	17	0	25
1 row	108	8	5	17	0	25
1 row	145	8	5	17	0	25
1 row	145	8	5	17	0	25
1 bar	230	7	4	10	5	280
1 bag	240	11	5	30	1	490
1 bag	240	8	5	33	1	790
8 chips	150	8	2	17	2	85
15 chips	140	8	3	17	3	138
⅓ bar	158	9	6	17	1	56
1 small handful	233	12	3	25	4	27
1 bar	140	5	0.5	19	3	30
1 bar	150	6	1.5	19	3	30

SNACK FOODS

FOOD	GI	LOW MED HIGH	SERVING SIZE
Granola Gourmet™ 4Real™ Energy Bar, Mocha Fudge	23	low	35 g
Granola Gourmet™ 4Real™ Energy Bar, Ultimate Berry	25	low	35 g
Gummi confectionary, based on glucose syrup	94	high	¾ oz
Jell-O, Raspberry flavor	53	low	4 oz
Jelly beans	78	high	¾ oz
Kudos Milk Chocolate Granola Bars, Peanut Butter Flavor	45	low	1 oz
Licorice, soft	78	high	1 oz
Life Savers®, peppermint	70	high	½ oz
Luna Protein Chocolate Peanut Butter Bar	28	low	1½ oz
Luna Cookie Dough Bar	18	low	1½ oz
Mars Bar®, regular	62	med	1 oz
Marshmallows, plain, pink, and white	62	med	½ oz
Milky Bar®, white, Nestlé®	44	low	1 oz
Milky Way Bar	62	med	2 oz
M&M's®, peanut	33	low	1 oz
Muesli bar, chewy, with chocolate chips or fruit	54	low	1 oz
Muesli bar, crunchy, with dried fruit	61	med	¾ oz
Nuts, mixed, roasted and salted	24	low	½ oz

@ part of GI symbol program   ★ little or no carbs

HOUSEHOLD MEASURE	CALORIES	FAT (g)	SATURATED FAT (g)	CARBO-HYDRATE (g)	FIBER (g)	SODIUM (mg)
1 bar	150	6	1.5	19	3	35
1 bar	150	6	0.5	19	3	20
5 pieces	63	0	0	15	0	3
½ cup	80	0	0	18	0	6
6 pieces	62	0	0	15	0	25
1 bar	130	6	3	17	1	75
2 pieces	61	0	0	14	1	31
¾ roll	65	0	0	16	0	1
1 bar	190	9	4	19	2	210
1 bar	180	6	4	21	3	230
1 fun-size bar	114	4	3	18	0	37
4 round pieces	48	0	0	15	0	5
2 mini-bars	168	10	6	17	0	35
1 bar	260	10	7	40	1	95
½ packet	142	8	3	17	0	15
¾ bar	98	3	1	15	0	60
1 bar	85	2	0	14	0	64
1 tbsp	84	7	1	4	1	95

SNACK FOODS

FOOD	GI	LOW MED HIGH	SERVING SIZE
Peanut Butter Chocolate Buddy™ bar, Revival Soy®	52	low	1 bar
Peanuts, roasted, salted	14	low	5½ oz
Performance Chocolate energy bar, Power Bar	53	low	2.2 oz
Pirate's Booty®, Aged White Cheddar snack	70	high	1 oz
Popcorn, plain, cooked in microwave	72	high	1 oz
Potato chips, plain, salted	57	med	1¾ oz
PowerBar®, Chocolate	53	low	2 oz
President's Choice® Blue Menu™ Chewy Cranberry Apple Granola Bar	58	med	0.9 oz
President's Choice® Blue Menu™ Flaxseed Tortilla Chips, Sea Salt	64	med	1¾ oz
President's Choice® Blue Menu™ Microwave Popping Corn, butter flavor	72	high	1½ oz
President's Choice® Blue Menu™ Microwave Popping Corn, natural flavor	58	med	1½ oz
President's Choice® Blue Menu™ Raspberry Fruit Bar, Fat-Free	74	high	1.35 oz
Pretzels, oven-baked, traditional wheat flavor	83	high	¾ oz
Rice Krispie Treat® bar, Kellogg's®	63	med	¾ oz

@ part of GI symbol program   ★ little or no carbs

HOUSEHOLD MEASURE	CALORIES	FAT (g)	SATURATED FAT (g)	CARBO-HYDRATE (g)	FIBER (g)	SODIUM (mg)
1 bar	260	7	1	30	5	320
1 cup	871	72	8	14	13	900
1 bar	230	2	1	44	4	200
1 package	130	5	1	19	0	140
3 cups	89	1	0	14	6	1
30 chips	271	19	5	27	2	260
1 bar	230	2	1	40	4	200
1 bar	100	2	0	21	1	55
17 chips	250	14	2	20	6	170
6 cups popped	160	3	1	31	5	230
6 cups popped	160	3	1	31	5	230
2 bars	130	0	0	32	1	105
1 small packet	76	1	0	13	1	396
1 bar	91	2	1	17	0	81

SNACK FOODS

FOOD	GI	LOW MED HIGH	SERVING SIZE
Roll-Ups®, processed fruit snack	99	high	¾ oz
Shaklee™ 180 Blueberry and Almond Crisp Meal-in-a-Bar	25	low	70 g
Shaklee™ 180 Crunch Peanut Butter Snack Bar	22	low	31 g
Shaklee™ 180 Peanut Butter and Chocolate Chip Crisp Meal-in-a-Bar	29	low	70 g
Skittles®	70	high	¾ oz
Snickers® Bar	43	low	2 oz
Snickers® Marathon Nutrition Bar, Dark Chocolate Crunch flavor	49	low	1.4 oz
Snickers® Marathon Nutrition Bar, Honey & Toasted Almond flavor	41	low	1.4 oz
Snickers® Marathon Protein Performance Bar, Caramel Nut Rush flavor	26	low	2¾ oz
Snickers® Marathon Protein Performance Bar, Chocolatey Nut Burst	32	low	2¾ oz
SoLo GI Energy Bar Apple Cinnamon 50g (Canada only)	35	low	50 g
SoLo GI Energy Bar Berry Bliss 50g (USA only)	29	low	50 g
SoLo GI Energy Bar Chocolate Charger 50g (USA and Canada)	28	low	50 g

@ part of GI symbol program ★ little or no carbs

HOUSEHOLD MEASURE	CALORIES	FAT (g)	SATURATED FAT (g)	CARBO-HYDRATE (g)	FIBER (g)	SODIUM (mg)
1	66	1	0	14	0	1
1 bar	260	6	1	32	6	400
1 bar	130	3	1	15	3	190
1 bar	270	7	3	32	6	400
5 pieces	82	1	1	18	0	9
1 bar	280	14	5	34	1	140
1 bar	150	5	3	15	7	140
1 bar	150	5	2	15	7	125
1 bar	290	10	5	30	10	190
1 bar	280	9	3	26	11	340
1 bar	200	6	2.5	27	3	125
1 bar	200	6	2.5	25	3	125
1 bar	200	7	3	26	4	120

SNACK FOODS

FOOD	GI	LOW MED HIGH	SERVING SIZE
SoLo GI Energy Bar Dark Chocolate Almond 50g (Canada only)	31	low	50 g
SoLo GI Energy Bar Dark Chocolate Mandarin 50g (Canada only)	30	low	50 g
SoLo GI Energy Bar Lemon Lift 50g (USA and Canada)	29	low	50 g
SoLo GI Energy Bar Mint Mania 50g (USA only)	23	low	50 g
SoLo GI Energy Bar Mocha Fudge 50g (Canada only)	32	low	50 g
SoLo GI Energy Bar Peanut Power 50g (USA and Canada)	27	low	50 g
SoLo GI Energy Bar Pineapple Coconut 50g (Canada only)	29	low	50 g
Stretch Island Fruit Co™ Summer Strawberry fruit leather	29	low	½ oz
Taste of Nature Argentina Peanut Plains Fruit and Nut Bar	21	low	1 bar
Taste of Nature Brazilian Nut Fiesta Fruit and Nut Bar	39	low	1 bar
Taste of Nature California Almond Valley Fruit and Nut Bar	41	low	1 bar
Taste of Nature Canadian Maple Forest Fruit and Nut Bar	37	low	1 bar
Taste of Nature Caribbean Ginger Island Fruit and Nut Bar	49	low	1 bar

@ part of GI symbol program   ★ little or no carbs

HOUSEHOLD MEASURE	CALORIES	FAT (g)	SATURATED FAT (g)	CARBO-HYDRATE (g)	FIBER (g)	SODIUM (mg)
1 bar	200	8	3	25	4	85
1 bar	190	7	3.5	27	3	95
1 bar	200	6	2.5	26	4	105
1 bar	200	7	3	26	4	120
1 bar	200	8	3.5	26	4	95
1 bar	200	8	3	23	3	125
1 bar	200	8	4	26	4	105
1 bar	45	0	0	11	1	0
40 g	220	17	3	12	3	45
40 g	190	12	2	17	2	5
40 g	180	11	2	18	3	10
40 g	190	12	2	19	3	35
40 g	180	9	1	21	2	10

SNACK FOODS

FOOD	GI	LOW MED HIGH	SERVING SIZE
Taste of Nature Himalayan Goji Summit Fruit and Nut Bar	38	low	1 bar
Taste of Nature Mediterranean Pistachio Passion Fruit and Nut Bar	43	low	1 bar
Taste of Nature Niagara Apple Country Fruit and Nut Bar	48	low	1 bar
Taste of Nature Nova Scotia Blueberry Fields Fruit and Nut Bar	44	low	1 bar
Taste of Nature Persian Pomegranate Garden Fruit and Nut Bar	52	low	1 bar
Taste of Nature Quebec Cranberry Carnival Fruit and Nut Bar	48	low	1 bar
Twisties®, cheese-flavored snack	74	high	1 oz
Twix® bar	44	low	½ oz
VO2 Max Chocolate Energy Bar, M&M/Mars	49	low	2.2 oz

@ part of GI symbol program   ★ little or no carbs

HOUSEHOLD MEASURE	CALORIES	FAT (g)	SATURATED FAT (g)	CARBO-HYDRATE (g)	FIBER (g)	SODIUM (mg)
40 g	180	11	2	17	5	5
40 g	180	10	1	21	3	50
40 g	150	5	1	25	3	10
40 g	150	10	1	20	4	5
40 g	160	8	1	21	3	5
40 g	180	11	2	19	3	10
½ oz packet	108	7	4	15	1	278
1 fun-size bar	91	5	3	12	1	28
1 bar	210	3	1	45	2	220

SOUPS

FOOD	GI	LOW MED HIGH	SERVING SIZE
Black bean, canned	64	med	8 oz
Chicken and mushroom soup	58	med	8 oz
Clear consommé, chicken or vegetable	★		8 fl oz
Green pea, canned	66	med	9 oz
Lentil, canned	44	low	9 oz
Minestrone, traditional	39	low	9 oz
Campbell's® Minestrone, condensed, prepared with water	48	low	8 oz
President's Choice® Blue Menu™ Chicken & Rotini Soup	38	low	9 oz
President's Choice® Blue Menu™ Lentil Soup	56	med	9 oz
President's Choice® Blue Menu™ Minestrone & Pasta Instant Soup, Low Fat	54	low	9 oz
President's Choice® Blue Menu™ Mushroom Barley, Ready-to-Serve	45	low	9 oz
President's Choice® Blue Menu™ Pasta e Fagioli Soup, Ready-to-Serve	52	low	9 oz
President's Choice® Blue Menu™ Spicy Black Bean Low Fat Instant Soup	57	med	9 oz

@ part of GI symbol program   ★ little or no carbs

HOUSEHOLD MEASURE	CALORIES	FAT (g)	SATURATED FAT (g)	CARBO-HYDRATE (g)	FIBER (g)	SODIUM (mg)
1 cup	108	1	0	18	4	1105
1 cup	274	18	5	18	1	1940
1 cup	17	0	0	2	0	1600
½ can	180	7	4	19	5	613
1 cup	98	1	0	13	5	867
1 cup	140	4	1	13	10	520
1 cup	180	2	1	28	6	1920
1 container	100	2	1	11	4	480
1 container	140	3	1	19	4	480
1 container	230	2	1	46	5	540
1 container	80	2	0	9	3	480
1 container	160	3	1	22	3	480
1 container	240	1	0	32	13	680

SOUPS

FOOD	GI	LOW MED HIGH	SERVING SIZE
President's Choice® Blue Menu™ Spicy Black Bean with Vegetables Soup	46	low	9 oz
President's Choice® Blue Menu™ Vegetarian Chili, Ready-to-Serve	39	low	9 oz
President's Choice® Blue Menu™ Vegetarian Chili Low Fat Instant Cup	36	low	9 oz
Pumpkin, Creamy, Heinz®	76	high	7 oz
Split pea, canned	60	med	8 oz
Tomato, canned	38	low	9 oz
Tomato soup, condensed, prepared with water, Campbell's®	52	low	8 oz
Vegetable soup	60	med	8 oz

@ part of GI symbol program   ★ little or no carbs

HOUSEHOLD MEASURE	CALORIES	FAT (g)	SATURATED FAT (g)	CARBO-HYDRATE (g)	FIBER (g)	SODIUM (mg)
1 container	200	3	0	34	7	480
1 container	200	3	1	29	5	480
1 container	230	2	0	29	11	420
½ can	106	2	0	16	4	672
1 cup	160	2	0	27	4	373
1 cup	70	1	0	14	3	850
1 cup	180	0	0	40	2	1420
1 cup	125	4	1	18	1	880

SOY PRODUCTS

FOOD	GI	LOW MED HIGH	SERVING SIZE
Flaxseed and soy bread	55	low	3 oz
President's Choice® Blue Menu™ Soy Beverage, Chocolate flavored	40	low	8 fl oz
President's Choice® Blue Menu™ Soy Beverage, Original flavored	15	low	8 fl oz
President's Choice® Blue Menu™ Soy Beverage, Vanilla flavored	28	low	8 fl oz
Soy beans, canned, drained	14	low	6 oz
Soy beans, dried, boiled	18	low	6 oz
Soy yogurt, Peach and Mango, 2% fat, with sugar	50	low	3½ oz
Vitasoy® Organic soy milk	43	low	8 fl oz

ⓖ part of GI symbol program   ★ little or no carbs

HOUSEHOLD MEASURE	CALORIES	FAT (g)	SATURATED FAT (g)	CARBO-HYDRATE (g)	FIBER (g)	SODIUM (mg)
2 slices	230	8	1	26	6	364
1 cup	160	3	1	28	0	140
1 cup	90	3	1	9	0	150
1 cup	120	3	1	16	0	160
1 cup	169	9	1	5	8	629
1 cup	242	13	2	2	12	15
½ container	69	2	0	8	1	58
1 cup	120	4	1	16	3	30

SPREADS & SWEETENERS

FOOD	GI	LOW MED HIGH	SERVING SIZE
100% Fruit Jam Apricot	50	low	1 oz
100% Fruit Jam Blackberry	46	low	1 oz
100% Fruit Jam Breakfast Marmalade	55	low	1 oz
100% Fruit Jam Raspberry	46	low	1 oz
100% Fruit Jam Strawberry	46	low	1 oz
Agave Syrup, Light Premium (IIDEA)	22.5	low	½ oz
Agave Syrup, Light Standard (IIDEA)	27.5	low	½ oz
Agave Syrup, Ragave	22	low	10 g
Anchovy fish paste	★		¾ oz
Apricot 100% Pure Fruit spread, no added sugar	43	low	½ oz
Apricot fruit spread, reduced sugar	55	low	½ oz
Butter	★		⅓ oz
Cashew spread	★		⅓ oz
Dairy blend, with canola oil	★		⅓ oz
Extra virgin olive oil spread	★		¼ oz
Fructose, pure	19	low	½ oz
Ginger Marmalade, original	50	low	¾ oz
Glucose tablets or powder	100	high	½ oz
Glucose syrup	100	high	¾ oz
Golden syrup	63	med	¾ oz

@ part of GI symbol program   ★ little or no carbs

HOUSEHOLD MEASURE	CALORIES	FAT (g)	SATURATED FAT (g)	CARBO-HYDRATE (g)	FIBER (g)	SODIUM (mg)
1 tbsp	64	0	0	15	0	3
1 tbsp	66	0	0	15	0	3
1 tbsp	68	0	0	17	0	3
1 tbsp	66	0	0	15	0	3
1 tbsp	65	0	0	15	0	3
1 tbsp	25	0	0	6	0	0
1 tbsp	25	0	0	6	0	0
1 tbsp	30	0	0	6	0	0
1 tbsp	4	2	1	1	0	240
1 tbsp	38	0	0	9	0	2
1 tbsp	20	0	0	6	0	10
2 tsp	0	9	6	0	0	78
2 tsp	2	5	1	3	1	2
2 tsp	0	8	4	0	0	52
1 tsp	0	4	1	0	0	18
3 tsp	61	0	0	15	0	0
2 tsp	56	0	0	14	0	2
1 tbsp	59	0	0	15	0	2
3 tsp	65	0	0	16	0	29
3 tsp	58	0	0	15	0	26

209

SPREADS & SWEETENERS

FOOD	GI	LOW MED HIGH	SERVING SIZE
Honey, Capilano, blended	64	med	¾ oz
Honey, general	55	low	¾ oz
Honey, Ironbark	48	low	¾ oz
Honey, Red Gum	46	low	¾ oz
Honey, Salvation Jane	64	med	¾ oz
Honey, Stringybark	44	low	¾ oz
Honey, Yapunya	52	low	¾ oz
Honey, Yellow-box	35	low	¾ oz
Hummus (chickpea dip)	22	low	1 oz
Jam, sweetened with aspartame	★		⅓ oz
Jam, sweetened with sucralose	★		⅓ oz
Jelly, grape	52	low	½ oz
Lemon butter, homemade	★		⅓ oz
Maple syrup, pure, Canadian	54	low	¾ oz
Margarine, canola	★		⅓ oz
Marmalade, orange	48	low	½ oz
Marmalade, sweetened with aspartame	★		⅓ oz
Marmalade, sweetened with sucralose	★		⅓ oz
Nutella®, hazelnut spread	25	low	1 oz
@ Premium Agave Nectar, Sweet Cactus Farms	19	low	¾ oz
President's Choice® Blue Menu™ Twice the Fruit Spread—Apricot	49	low	½ oz

@ part of GI symbol program   ★ little or no carbs

HOUSEHOLD MEASURE	CALORIES	FAT (g)	SATURATED FAT (g)	CARBO-HYDRATE (g)	FIBER (g)	SODIUM (mg)
3 tsp	70	0	0	18	0	3
3 tsp	70	0	0	18	0	3
3 tsp	70	0	0	18	0	3
3 tsp	70	0	0	18	0	3
3 tsp	70	0	0	18	0	3
3 tsp	70	0	0	18	0	3
3 tsp	0	0	0	18	0	3
3 tsp	0	0	0	18	0	3
1½ tbsp	73	5	1	6	3	93
2 tsp	0	0	0	0	0	8
2 tsp	0	0	0	0	0	8
1 packet	42	0	0	10	0	5
2 tsp	1	2	1	3	0	18
3 tsp	52	0	0	13	0	2
2 tsp	0	7	1	0	0	79
1 tbsp	37	0	0	13	0	11
2 tsp	0	0	0	0	0	3
2 tsp	0	0	0	0	0	3
1½ tbsp	157	10	3	17	0	15
4 tsp	64	0	0	16	0	3
1 tbsp	25	0	0	6	0	2

SPREADS & SWEETENERS

FOOD	GI	LOW MED HIGH	SERVING SIZE
President's Choice® Blue Menu™ Twice the Fruit Spread—Strawberry & Rhubarb	69	med	½ oz
St. Dalfour's Black Cherry Jam	50	low	1 oz
St. Dalfour's Mirabelle Plum Jam	54	low	1 oz
St. Dalfour's Orange Marmalade	54	low	1 oz
St. Dalfour's Red Raspberry Jam	55	low	1 oz
St. Dalfour's Royal Fig Jam	51	low	1 oz
St. Dalfour's Strawberry Jam	52	low	1 oz
St. Dalfour's Thick Apricot Jam	54	low	1 oz
St. Dalfour's Wild Blueberry Jam	52	low	1 oz
Strawberry jam, regular	51	low	¾ oz
Sugar, brown	61	med	½ oz
Sugar, white	65	med	5 g
Tahini	★		¾ oz

ⓖ part of GI symbol program   ★ little or no carbs

HOUSEHOLD MEASURE	CALORIES	FAT (g)	SATURATED FAT (g)	CARBO-HYDRATE (g)	FIBER (g)	SODIUM (mg)
1 tbsp	25	0	0	6	0	0
1 tbsp	56	0	0	13	0	0
1 tbsp	56	0	0	13	0	0
1 tbsp	56	0	0	14	0	0
1 tbsp	56	0	0	14	0	0
1 tbsp	56	0	0	13	0	0
1 tbsp	56	0	0	13	0	0
1 tbsp	56	0	0	13	0	0
1 tbsp	56	0	0	13	0	0
3 tsp	53	0	0	13	0	3
6 tsp	65	0	0	17	0	5
1 tsp	15	0	0	4	0	0
1 tbsp	4	12	2	0	0	16

Nutritive Sweeteners

Fructose

GI 19 4 cal per gram 11 cal per teaspoon table sugar equivalent*	Fructose or fruit sugar has a relatively small effect on blood glucose levels. It is sweeter than table sugar, but has the same number of calories per gram. Sweetness relative to table sugar = up to 70% more, depending on the temperature of the food

Glucose

GI 100 4 cal per gram 26 cal per teaspoon table sugar equivalent*	Glucose is the sugar found in blood. When eaten, it causes blood glucose levels to rise rapidly. It is not as sweet as table sugar, but has the same number of calories per gram. Sweetness relative to table sugar = 25% less

Golden syrup

GI 63 3 cal per gram 11 cal per teaspoon table sugar equivalent*	Golden syrup has a moderate effect on blood glucose levels, very similar to table sugar. It is sweeter than table sugar, and has fewer calories per gram. Sweetness relative to table sugar = 33% more

* The number of calories in the volume of alternative sweetener that provides the equivalent sweetness to 1 teaspoon of table sugar.

Nutritive Sweeteners

Grape syrup

GI 52

4 cal per gram

16 cal per teaspoon
table sugar equivalent*

Grape syrup or nectar has a moderate effect on blood glucose levels. It is a little sweeter than table sugar, but has the same number of calories.

Sweetness relative to table sugar = 20% more

Honey

GI 35–64

4 cal per gram

20 cal per teaspoon
table sugar equivalent*

Honey has a variable effect on blood glucose levels depending on whether it is a blend or a pure floral honey. The pure floral honeys appear to have lower GIs. On average, honey is slightly less sweet than table sugar, but has about the same number of calories per teaspoon.

Sweetness relative to table sugar = about the same

Isomalt

GI 60

3 cal per gram

26 cal per teaspoon
table sugar equivalent*

Isomalt has a moderate effect on blood glucose levels similar to table sugar. It is only half as sweet as table sugar, but has fewer calories, and may have a laxative effect if eaten in large quantities.

Sweetness relative to table sugar = half as sweet

Nutritive Sweeteners

Lactose

GI 46

4 cal per gram

120 cal per teaspoon
table sugar equivalent*

Lactose is the sugar found in milk. It causes blood glucose levels to rise slowly. It is not very sweet at all, but has the same number of calories as table sugar.

Sweetness relative to table sugar = 85% less sweet

Maltitol

GI 69

3 cal per gram

21 cal per teaspoon
table sugar equivalent*

Maltitol has a moderate to high effect on blood glucose levels greater than that of table sugar. It is only three-quarters as sweet as table sugar, and has the same number of calories, and may have a laxative effect and cause flatulence and diarrhea if eaten in large quantities.

Sweetness relative to table sugar = 25% less sweet

Maltodextrin

GI not known

4 cal per gram

35 cal per teaspoon
table sugar equivalent*

Maltodextrins are short chain glucose polymers with a GI similar to that of glucose. They are only half as sweet as table sugar, and have the same number of calories.

Sweetness relative to table sugar = half as sweet

* The number of calories in the volume of alternative sweetener that provides the equivalent sweetness to 1 teaspoon of table sugar.

Nutritive Sweeteners

Maltose

GI 105

4 cal per gram

60 cal per teaspoon
table sugar equivalent*

Maltose or malt causes blood glucose levels to rise rapidly. It is only one-third as sweet as table sugar, and has the same number of calories.

Sweetness relative to table sugar = 67% less sweet

Mannitol

GI n/a

2 cal per gram

15 cal per teaspoon
table sugar equivalent*

Mannitol has essentially no effect on blood glucose levels. It is only three-quarters as sweet as table sugar, but has only half the amount of calories, and may have a laxative effect and cause gas and diarrhea if eaten in large quantities.

Sweetness relative to table sugar = 25% less sweet

Maple syrup

GI 54

3 cal per gram

15 cal per teaspoon
table sugar equivalent*

Pure maple syrup has a moderate effect on blood glucose levels. It is a little sweeter than table sugar, but has fewer calories.
Sweetness relative to table sugar = 10% more

Nutritive Sweeteners

Polydextrose

GI 7

1 cal per gram

6 cal per teaspoon
table sugar equivalent*

Polydextrose has very little effect on blood glucose levels. It is not sweet, but is used as a bulking agent with nonnutritive sweeteners. It has only one-third the amount of calories as table sugar, but may have a laxative effect if eaten in large quantities.

Sweetness relative to table sugar = not sweet

Table sugar (sucrose)

GI 60 (average)

4 cal per gram

16 cal per teaspoon

Sucrose or table sugar is the most common sweetener eaten in North America. Despite popular misconceptions, it causes blood glucose levels to rise only moderately (less than white bread).

Sweetness = 100%
Castor sugar, brown sugar, raw sugar, confectioners' sugar are all forms of sugar.

Xylitol

GI 21

3 cal per gram

14 cal per teaspoon
table sugar equivalent*

Xylitol is a sugar alcohol that has little effect on blood glucose levels. It is as sweet as sugar and has fewer calories, but may have a laxative effect and cause gas and diarrhea if consumed in large quantities. Sweetness relative to table sugar = 100% as sweet

* The number of calories in the volume of alternative sweetener that provides the equivalent sweetness to 1 teaspoon of table sugar.

Nonnutritive Sweeteners

Acesulphame potassium or Acesulphame K

GI 0	Acesulphame K is much sweeter than sugar, has no effect on blood glucose levels, and doesn't provide any calories because it is not absorbed into the body.
0 cal per gram	
0 cal per teaspoon table sugar equivalent*	
Food additive code 950	
Brand names: Sweet One, Sunett	Sweetness relative to table sugar = 200 times more

Aspartame

GI 0	Aspartame is a couple of hundred times sweeter than sugar, and has essentially no effect on blood glucose levels. Because it is a protein, it does provide some calories, but because it is very sweet, you only use it in small amounts.
4 cal per gram	
0.3 cal per teaspoon table sugar equivalent*	
Brand names: Nutrasweet, Equal, Equal Spoonful	
	Sweetness relative to table sugar = 150–250 times more
	Warning: Aspartame should not be used by people with phenylketonuria.

Nonnutritive Sweeteners

Neotame

GI 0

4 cal per gram

0 cal per teaspoon
table sugar equivalent*

Neotame is many thousands of times sweeter than sugar, and has essentially no effect on blood glucose levels. Because it is a protein, it does provide some calories, but because it is extremely sweet, it is only used in tiny amounts.

Sweetness relative to table sugar = 7,000–13,000 times more

While neotame is approved by the Food and Drug Administration (FDA), it is not currently found in many foods or beverages.

Saccharin

GI 0

0 cal per gram

0 cal per teaspoon
table sugar equivalent*

Brand names: Sweet'N Low, Sugar Twin

Saccharin is hundreds of times sweeter than sugar, has no effect on blood glucose levels, and is not metabolized by the human body.

Sweetness relative to table sugar = 300–500 times more

Stevia

GI 0

2.7 cal per gram

0.7 cal per teaspoon
table sugar equivalent*

Stevia is considerably sweeter than sugar and has essentially no effect on blood glucose levels.

Sweetness relative to table sugar = 30 times more

---

* The number of calories in the volume of alternative sweetener that provides the equivalent sweetness to 1 teaspoon of table sugar.

Nonnutritive Sweeteners

Sucralose

GI 0

0 cal per gram

0 cal per teaspoon
table sugar equivalent*

Brand name: Splenda

Sucralose is hundreds of times sweeter than sugar, has no effect on blood glucose levels, and does not provide any calories because it is not absorbed into the body.

Sweetness relative to table sugar = 400–600 times more

VEGETABLES

FOOD	GI	LOW MED HIGH	SERVING SIZE
Alfalfa sprouts	★		½ oz
Artichoke, globe	★		4 oz
Artichoke hearts, whole, canned	★		1½ oz
Artichokes in brine	★		1½ oz
Artichoke hearts in brine, drained	★		3 oz
Arugula	★		¾ oz
Asparagus	★		3 oz
Asparagus, canned, drained	★		3 oz
Asparagus green/white spears, canned	★		2 oz
Asparagus in springwater	★		2 oz
Baby corn, cut, canned	★		1¾ oz
Baby corn spears, whole, canned	★		1¾ oz
Bamboo shoots, canned	★		1 oz
Bean sprouts, cooked	★		2 oz
Bean sprouts, raw	★		1 oz
Beans, green	★		1¾ oz
Beans, Chinese long	★		2½ oz
Beets, canned	**64**	med	6 oz
Bok choy	★		3 oz
Broccoflower	★		1½ oz
Broccoli	★		3½ oz
Brussels sprouts	★		2¾ oz
Cabbage, Chinese	★		3 oz

@ part of GI symbol program   ★ little or no carbs

HOUSEHOLD MEASURE	CALORIES	FAT (g)	SATURATED FAT (g)	CARBO-HYDRATE (g)	FIBER (g)	SODIUM (mg)
6 tbsp	4	0	0	0	0	7
1 medium	28	0	0	2	1	7
1 heart	14	0	0	1	0	80
1 heart	12	0	0	2	0	130
2 hearts	19	0	0	1	2	249
3 medium leaves	6	0	0	1	0	6
8 small spears	20	0	0	1	1	2
¾ cup	22	0	0	1	4	216
½ cup	12	0	0	1	0	104
½ cup	8	0	0	1	0	110
⅓ cup	13	0	0	2	1	135
⅓ cup	13	0	0	2	1	105
¼ cup	4	0	0	0	1	3
½ cup	16	0	0	1	2	1
⅓ cup	6	0	0	0	0	69
10 beans	14	0	0	1	2	2
½ cup	21	0	0	1	3	1
1 cup sliced	82	0	0	16	5	540
½ cup	30	2	1	1	1	21
½ cup	13	0	0	1	1	8
1 cup	34	0	0	1	4	20
4 sprouts	25	0	0	2	3	23
½ cup	29	2	1	1	1	18

VEGETABLES

FOOD	GI	LOW MED HIGH	SERVING SIZE
Cabbage, green, cooked	★		3 oz
Cabbage, green, raw	★		3 oz
Cabbage, red, cooked	★		3 oz
Cabbage, red, raw	★		3 oz
Carrots, peeled, boiled	39	low	3 oz
Cauliflower	★		3 oz
Celery, cooked	★		2½ oz
Celery, raw	★		1 oz
Chili, banana, cooked	★		1¾ oz
Chili, banana, raw	★		2 oz
Chili, hot thin, cooked	★		¾ oz
Chili, hot thin, raw	★		1 oz
Chives	★		¼ oz
Chayote	★		1½ oz
Cucumber	★		1 oz
Cucumber, Persian	★		1 oz
Eggplant, cooked	★		1¾ oz
Eggplant, raw	★		1½ oz
Endive	★		3 oz
Fennel, cooked	★		2½ oz
Fennel, raw	★		1¾ oz
Garlic	★		¼ oz
Ginger	★		⅒ oz

@ part of GI symbol program   ★ little or no carbs

HOUSEHOLD MEASURE	CALORIES	FAT (g)	SATURATED FAT (g)	CARBO-HYDRATE (g)	FIBER (g)	SODIUM (mg)
½ cup	20	0	0	2	3	15
1 cup	23	0	0	2	3	17
½ cup	26	0	0	3	3	14
1 cup	30	0	0	3	4	15
½ cup	30	0	0	6	2	49
¾ cup	21	0	0	2	2	13
2 medium stalks	13	0	0	2	2	63
2 small stalks	5	0	0	1	1	28
1 average	10	0	0	1	1	2
1 average	10	0	0	1	1	2
1 average	6	0	0	1	1	1
1 average	9	0	0	1	1	1
1 tbsp	1	0	0	0	0	0
¼ average	9	0	0	2	1	3
3 slices	3	0	0	0	0	5
3 slices	4	0	0	1	0	5
1 slice	12	0	0	1	1	2
½ cup	9	0	0	1	1	2
½ cup	16	0	0	0	2	81
½ cup	20	0	0	3	3	26
½ cup	12	0	0	2	1	19
1 clove	4	0	0	0	1	0
1 tsp	0	0	0	0	0	0

VEGETABLES

FOOD	GI	LOW MED HIGH	SERVING SIZE
Green beans, sliced, canned	★		3 oz
Green plantain, peeled, boiled, 10 mins	39	low	4 oz
Green plantain, peeled, fried in vegetable oil	40	low	4 oz
Hash browns	75	high	2 oz
Herbs, fresh or dried	★		1/10 oz
Horseradish	★		1/4 oz
Kohlrabi	★		3 oz
Leeks, cooked	★		3 oz
Leeks, raw	★		3 oz
Lettuce, cos	★		3/4 oz
Lettuce, iceberg	★		3/4 oz
Lettuce, Boston Bibb	★		3/4 oz
Mashed potato, made with milk	85	high	4 oz
Mashed potato, made with milk and margarine	71	high	4.2 oz
Mixed vegetables, Chinese, canned	★		3 oz
Mushrooms	★		1 1/4 oz
Mushrooms, canned	★		1 oz
Mushrooms, shiitake, canned	★		1 oz
Okra	★		3 oz
Onion	★		1 oz
Onions, canned, sautéed and diced	★		1 3/4 oz

ⓖ part of GI symbol program   ★ little or no carbs

HOUSEHOLD MEASURE	CALORIES	FAT (g)	SATURATED FAT (g)	CARBO- HYDRATE (g)	FIBER (g)	SODIUM (mg)
⅓ cup	30	0	0	5	3	281
½ cup	150	1	0	37	3	5
½ cup	194	6	1	37	3	5
1 average square	171	12	5	15	1	281
1 tsp	0	0	0	0	0	0
1 average	4	0	0	1	0	0
½ cup	36	0	0	4	3	12
1 average	27	0	0	3	2	13
1 average	28	0	0	3	3	14
3 medium leaves	5	0	0	0	1	4
3 medium leaves	2	0	0	0	0	5
3 medium leaves	4	0	0	0	1	4
½ cup	82	1	0	15	2	10
½ cup	117	4	1	20	2	350
⅓ cup	26	0	0	5	1	68
½ cup	11	0	0	1	1	3
3 small	11	1	0	1	1	5
3 small	8	0	0	1	1	96
½ cup	29	0	0	1	4	2
½ medium	13	0	0	2	1	4
1 medium	26	1	0	3	1	215

VEGETABLES

FOOD	GI	LOW MED HIGH	SERVING SIZE
Onions, sautèed and diced	★		½ oz
Parsley, cooked	★		1½ oz
Parsley, raw	★		¼ oz
Parsnips, boiled	52	low	2¾ oz
Peas, green	51	low	7 oz
Pepper, green, canned	★		1½ oz
Pepper, green, raw	★		1½ oz
Pepper, red, canned	★		1½ oz
Pepper, red, cooked	★		1½ oz
Potato, baked, without skin	85	high	3½ oz
Potato, Carisma, unpeeled, boiled 8 mins (or until al dente), Coles	53	low	4 oz
Potato chips, deep-fried	75	high	1½ oz
Potatoes, Baked, Russet Burbank potatoes, baked, without fat	85	high	5.75 oz
Potatoes, boiled	59	med	5.75 oz
Potatoes, Désirée, red-skinned type, peeled, boiled 35 mins	101	high	4 oz
Potato, instant, mashed, Idahoan	97	high	4 oz
Potatoes, Nardine, peeled, boiled	70	high	4 oz
Potatoes, new, canned, microwaved 3 mins	65	med	5 oz

HOUSEHOLD MEASURE	CALORIES	FAT (g)	SATURATED FAT (g)	CARBO-HYDRATE (g)	FIBER (g)	SODIUM (mg)
1 medium slice	6	0	0	1	0	2
½ cup	10	0	0	0	2	21
1 tbsp	1	0	0	0	0	2
½ cup	16	0	0	8	1	1
1½ cups	128	0	0	15	13	2
¼ cup	8	0	0	1	0	1
4 rings	7	0	0	1	0	1
¼ cup	12	0	0	2	1	0
4 rings	11	0	0	2	1	0
1 medium	72	0	0	14	1	8
1 medium	113	<1	<1	22	2	33
10 average chips	126	7	3	14	1	72
1 med potato	168	0	0	41	4	24
1 med potato	144	0	0	36	3	8
1 medium (2¾-inch diameter)	82	0	0	16	2	4
½ cup, prepared	170	0	0	16	2	15
1 medium (2¾-inch diameter)	82	0	0	16	2	4
4 small (1-inch diameter)	84	0	0	16	2	470

VEGETABLES

FOOD	GI	LOW MED HIGH	SERVING SIZE
Potatoes, new, unpeeled, boiled 20 mins	78	high	5 oz
Potatoes, Ontario, white, baked in skin	60	med	5.75 oz
Potatoes, Pontiac, peeled, boiled 15 mins, mashed	91	high	4 oz
Potatoes, Pontiac, peeled, boiled whole 30–35 mins	72	high	4 oz
Potatoes, Pontiac, peeled, microwaved 7 mins	79	high	4 oz
Potatoes, red, boiled with skin on in salted water 12 mins	89	high	5.75 oz
Potato, red, cubed, boiled in salted water 12 mins, stored overnight in refrigerator, consumed cold	56	med	5.75 oz
Potatoes, Sebago, peeled, boiled 35 mins	87	high	4 oz
Potato, wedge, with skin	75	high	1¼ oz
Potato salad, canned	63	med	4 oz
Pumpkin, boiled	66	med	7½ oz
Radishes, red	★		2 oz
Rutabaga	72	high	5.75 oz
Sauerkraut, canned	★		2½ oz
Seaweed	★		1½ oz
Shallots, cooked	★		1 oz
Shallots, raw	★		½ oz
Snowpeas, cooked	★		2¾ oz

ⓖ part of GI symbol program   ★ little or no carbs

HOUSEHOLD MEASURE	CALORIES	FAT (g)	SATURATED FAT (g)	CARBO-HYDRATE (g)	FIBER (g)	SODIUM (mg)
4 small (1-inch diameter)	84	0	0	16	2	4
1 med potato	161	0	0	41	4	17
½ cup	74	0	0	14	2	4
1 medium (2¾-inch diameter)	82	0	0	16	2	4
1 medium (2¾-inch diameter)	82	0	0	16	2	4
1 med potato	148	0	0	37	3	7
1 med potato	148	0	0	37	3	7
1 medium (2¾-inch diameter)	82	0	0	16	2	4
2 small	118	4	1	17	2	23
½ cup	147	8	2	16	1	408
1¼ cup	96	1	1	15	3	2
6 large	9	0	0	1	1	12
1 cup sliced	66	0	0	18	3	34
½ cup	12	0	0	1	3	322
½ cup	13	0	0	0	5	60
3 medium	9	0	0	1	0	33
2 average	4	0	0	1	0	16
20 average	39	0	0	4	2	1

VEGETABLES

FOOD	GI	LOW MED HIGH	SERVING SIZE
Snowpeas, raw	★		1 oz
Spinach, cooked	★		3 oz
Spinach, raw	★		1 oz
Spring onions	★		½ oz
Squash	★		2½ oz
Squash, butternut, boiled	51	low	2¾ oz
Sweet corn, Honey 'n Pearl variety, boiled	37	low	2¾ oz
Sweet corn, on the cob, boiled	48	low	2¾ oz
Sweet corn, whole kernel, canned, drained	46	low	3 oz
Sweet potato, baked	46	low	3 oz
Sweet potato, peeled, cubed, boiled in salted water 15 mins	59	med	5 oz
Swiss chard	★		4 oz
Taro, boiled	54	low	1½ oz
Tomatoes	★		1¾ oz
Tomatoes, in tomato juice	★		3 oz
Tomatoes, Italian diced	★		4½ oz
Tomatoes, Italian whole peeled Roma	★		4½ oz
Tomatoes, whole peeled, no added salt	★		4½ oz
Tomato, onion, pepper, celery	★		3 oz
Tomato puree	★		2 oz

@ part of GI symbol program   ★ little or no carbs

HOUSEHOLD MEASURE	CALORIES	FAT (g)	SATURATED FAT (g)	CARBO-HYDRATE (g)	FIBER (g)	SODIUM (mg)
10 average	12	0	0	2	1	0
⅔ cup	28	0	0	1	6	18
1 cup	6	0	0	0	1	6
1 medium	5	0	0	1	0	0
2 average	22	0	0	2	2	1
½ cup	30	0	0	6	2	2
1 medium (5 inches long)	84	1	0	15	2	6
1 medium (5 inches long)	84	1	0	15	2	6
½ cup	90	1	0	16	3	238
½ large	79	0	0	16	2	12
1 med potato	115	0	0	31	4	41
1 cup	24	0	0	2	4	213
½ cup	63	0	0	15	2	7
½ small	9	0	0	1	1	3
⅓ cup	19	0	0	3	1	56
½ cup	28	1	1	5	2	125
½ cup	30	1	1	5	2	125
½ cup	25	0	0	4	1	6
⅓ cup	19	0	0	3	1	60
¼ cup	20	0	0	3	1	221

VEGETABLES

FOOD	GI	LOW MED HIGH	SERVING SIZE
Turnips	★		1¾ oz
Water chestnuts, drained	★		¾ oz
Watercress	★		¼ oz
Yam, peeled, boiled	35	low	2½ oz
Zucchini, cooked	★		3 oz
Zucchini, raw	★		2 oz

@ part of GI symbol program   ★ little or no carbs

HOUSEHOLD MEASURE	CALORIES	FAT (g)	SATURATED FAT (g)	CARBO-HYDRATE (g)	FIBER (g)	SODIUM (mg)
⅓ cup	14	0	0	2	2	12
2 tbsp	11	0	0	2	1	2
¼ cup	1	0	0	0	0	3
½ cup	79	0	0	16	3	5
1 medium	17	0	0	2	2	1
½ medium	10	0	0	1	1	1

WEIGHT MANAGEMENT PRODUCTS

FOOD	GI	LOW MED HIGH	SERVING SIZE
BEVERAGES			
All Sport	53	low	8 fl oz
Arbonne Essentials® Chocolate Protein Shake Mix	27	low	45 g
Arbonne Essentials® Vanilla Protein Shake Mix	26	low	42 g
Gatorade®	78	high	8 fl oz
Optifast VLCD Banana Shake	24	low	1.8 oz powder
Optifast VLCD Chocolate Shake	31	low	1.8 oz powder
Optifast VLCD Coffee Shake	31	low	1.8 oz powder
Optifast VLCD Strawberry Shake	27	low	1.8 oz powder
Optifast VLCD Vanilla Shake	27	low	1.8 oz powder
Slim Fast™ French Vanilla ready-to-drink shake	37	low	11 fl oz
Svelte Chocolate Protein Drink	21	low	15.9 fl oz
Svelte French Vanilla Protein Drink	24	low	15.9 fl oz

© part of GI symbol program   ★ little or no carbs

HOUSEHOLD MEASURE	CALORIES	FAT (g)	SATURATED FAT (g)	CARBO-HYDRATE (g)	FIBER (g)	SODIUM (mg)
1 cup	60	0	0	16	0	55
2 scoops	160	3.5	0	15	2	480
2 scoops	160	3	0	14	1	360
1 cup	63	0	0	15	0	118
1 packet (without milk added)	207	4.5	1	23	4	220
1 packet (without milk added)	207	4.5	1	23	4	220
1 packet (without milk added)	207	4.5	1	23	4	220
1 packet (without milk added)	207	4.5	1	23	4	220
1 packet (without milk added)	207	4.5	1	23	4	220
1 can	220	3	1	35	5	220
1 pkg	260	10	2	35	5	190
1 pkg	260	10	1.5	35	5	190

WEIGHT MANAGEMENT PRODUCTS

FOOD	GI	LOW MED HIGH	SERVING SIZE
CAKES & MUFFINS			
Nutrisystem® Apple Strudel Scone	44	low	1 scone
Nutrisystem® Chocolate Cake	53	low	1 cake
Nutrisystem® Chocolate Frosted Donut	54	low	1 donut
Nutrisystem® Cranberry Orange Pastry	28	low	1 pastry
Nutrisystem® Double Chocolate Muffin	56	med	1 muffin
Nutrisystem® Golden Pound Cake	52	low	1 cake
MEALS, PREPARED & CONVENIENCE			
Nutrisystem® Apple Cinnamon Oatmeal	42	low	1 packet
Nutrisystem® Beef & Wedged Potatoes	38	low	1 container
Nutrisystem® Black Beans and Rice	68	med	1 container
Nutrisystem® Butternut Squash Ravioli	47	low	1 container
Nutrisystem® Cajun Style Chicken and Sausage	31	low	1 container
Nutrisystem® Cheese Tortellini	41	low	1 container
Nutrisystem® Cheesy Home-Style Potatoes	60	med	1 container
Nutrisystem® Chicken & Dumplings	32	low	1 container

@ part of GI symbol program   ★ little or no carbs

HOUSEHOLD MEASURE	CALORIES	FAT (g)	SATURATED FAT (g)	CARBO-HYDRATE (g)	FIBER (g)	SODIUM (mg)
1 scone	160	3	2	26	6	270
1 cake	160	5	1	24	5	250
1 donut	150	5	2	20	5	190
1 pastry	150	4	2	24	6	250
1 muffin	190	5	2	30	9	270
1 cake	160	5	1	24	5	250
1 packet	130	2	0	26	3	170
1 container	180	5	1	21	2	510
1 container	210	2	0	40	8	480
1 container	230	6	2	37	3	430
1 container	190	5	1	20	2	500
1 container	170	3	1	27	2	550
1 container	200	5	3	31	4	360
1 container	230	4	1	34	3	570

WEIGHT MANAGEMENT PRODUCTS

FOOD	GI	LOW MED HIGH	SERVING SIZE
Nutrisystem® Chicken Cacciatore Parmesan	27	low	I container
Nutrisystem® Chicken Fajita Melt	51	low	I package
Nutrisystem® Granola Cereal	48	low	I packet
NutriSystem® Hearty Beef Stew	26	low	I container
Nutrisystem® Honey Wheat Bagel	59	med	I bagel
Nutrisystem® Lasagna with Meat Sauce	26	low	I container
Nutrisystem® Maple Brown Sugar Oatmeal	62	med	I packet
Nutrisystem® Meatloaf & Mashed Potatoes	35	low	I container
Nutrisystem® Mexican Style Tortilla Soup	44	low	I container
Nutrisystem® Mushroom Risotto	52	low	I container
Nutrisystem® Pasta & Beef	33	low	I container
Nutrisystem® Ravioli in Basil Tomato Sauce	30	low	I container
Nutrisystem® Red Beans & Rice	44	low	I packet
Nutrisystem® Rotini & Meatballs	29	low	I container
Nutrisystem® Split Pea Soup	48	low	I container
Nutrisystem® Steak and Cheese Melt	45	low	I package
Nutrisystem® Sweet and Sour Chicken	44	low	I container

@ part of GI symbol program   ★ little or no carbs

HOUSEHOLD MEASURE	CALORIES	FAT (g)	SATURATED FAT (g)	CARBO-HYDRATE (g)	FIBER (g)	SODIUM (mg)
1 container	130	2	1	18	2	590
1 package	210	6	2	30	3	380
1 packet	160	3	0	31	3	90
1 container	150	3	1	16	1	510
1 bagel	170	2	1	33	4	250
1 container	280	8	4	33	3	590
1 packet	150	2	0	29	4	140
1 container	260	5	3	37	6	490
1 container	150	2	1	26	5	500
1 container	200	5	1	27	4	580
1 container	170	5	2	21	2	570
1 container	220	7	4	30	4	620
1 packet	170	3	1	31	5	530
1 container	220	6	3	26	3	600
1 container	170	1	0	31	9	560
1 package	230	8	3	29	4	510
1 container	260	3	1	38	2	570

WEIGHT MANAGEMENT PRODUCTS

FOOD	GI	LOW MED HIGH	SERVING SIZE
Nutrisystem® Three Cheese Chicken and Pasta	42	low	1 container
Nutrisystem® Turkey & Italian Sausage Pizza	65	med	1 pizza
Nutrisystem® Vegetable Lasagna	37	low	1 container
Nutrisystem® Wedding Soup	66	med	1 container
MEAL REPLACEMENTS			
Arbonne Essentials® Protein Shake Mix Meal Replacement—Chocolate	41	low	62 g
Arbonne Essentials® Protein Shake Mix Meal Replacement—Vanilla	48	low	60 g
Nutrimeal™ meal replacement drink, Usana	20	low	8 fl oz
SNACK FOODS			
Cinch™ Chocolate Decadence Bar	29	low	1 oz
Cinch™ Lemon Cranberry Bar	23	low	1 oz
Cinch™ Peanut Butter Bar	22	low	1 oz
ExtendBar™, Apple Cinnamon Delight Bar	33	low	1.35 oz
ExtendBar™, Chocolate Delight Bar	41	low	1.35 oz
ExtendBar™, Peanut Delight Bar	32	low	1.35 oz
Nutrisystem® Apple Granola Bar	52	low	1.4 oz
Nutrisystem® Butter Popcorn	34	low	1 package

ⓖ part of GI symbol program   ★ little or no carbs

HOUSEHOLD MEASURE	CALORIES	FAT (g)	SATURATED FAT (g)	CARBO-HYDRATE (g)	FIBER (g)	SODIUM (mg)
1 container	200	4	2	31	3	600
1 pizza	210	5	2	31	2	470
1 container	250	6	3	37	4	540
1 container	160	4	2	22	2	590
3 scoops	230	5	0.5	29	7	270
3 scoops	230	5	0.5	26	5	330
1 cup	163	5	1	17	6	189
1 bar	120	3	1	15	3	170
1 bar	120	3	1	15	3	150
1 bar	120	3	1	15	3	190
1 bar	150	2	0	21	5	135
1 bar	150	3	2	21	5	170
1 bar	150	3	1	21	5	160
1 bar	150	2	0	28	2	50
1 package	140	7	1	16	4	140

WEIGHT MANAGEMENT PRODUCTS

FOOD	GI	LOW MED HIGH	SERVING SIZE
Nutrisystem® Chewy Chocolate Chip Granola Bar	44	low	I bar
Nutrisystem® Chewy Peanut Bar	41	low	I bar
Nutrisystem® Chocolate Caramel Bar	48	low	I bar
Nutrisystem® Chocolate Chip Cookies	29	low	I package
Nutrisystem® Chocolate Chip Pudding Mix	26	low	I packet
Nutrisystem® Chocolate Crunch Bar	41	low	I oz
Nutrisystem® Chocolate Peanut Butter Bar (lunch)	20	low	I bar
Nutrisystem® Chocolatey Delight Bar	48	low	I bar
Nutrisystem® Chocolatey Nougat Bar	51	low	I bar
Nutrisystem® Fudge Bar	54	low	I bar
Nutrisystem® Fudge Brownie	54	low	I brownie
Nutrisystem® Fudge Graham Bar	66	med	I bar
Nutrisystem® Honey Mustard Pretzel Bits	32	low	I package
Nutrisystem® Ice Cream Sandwich	61	low	I sandwich
Nutrisystem® Nutrichocolates	29	low	I package
Nutrisystem® Peanut Butter Cookie	24	low	I cookie

@ part of GI symbol program   ★ little or no carbs

HOUSEHOLD MEASURE	CALORIES	FAT (g)	SATURATED FAT (g)	CARBO-HYDRATE (g)	FIBER (g)	SODIUM (mg)
1 bar	150	4	2	23	2	150
1 bar	180	8	3	21	5	115
1 bar	160	5	3	24	3	140
1 package	150	6	4	18	3	85
1 packet	60	2	1	14	4	100
1 container	130	6	5	15	0	130
1 bar	220	10	5	28	3	230
1 bar	140	4	3	23	5	70
1 bar	160	7	4	23	4	50
1 bar	90	1	1	18	4	90
1 brownie	170	6	1	24	9	300
1 bar	200	7	5	25	3	200
1 package	140	7	3	12	4	260
1 sandwich	130	2	1	25	3	130
1 package	150	8	7	13	1	35
1 cookie	160	7	2	20	4	180

WEIGHT MANAGEMENT PRODUCTS

FOOD	GI	LOW MED HIGH	SERVING SIZE
Nutrisystem® Peanut Butter Granola Bar	32	med	1 bar
Nutrisystem® Peppermint Cookie Patty	36	low	1 patty
Nutrisystem® Pretzels	57	low	1 package
Nutrisystem® Thin Mint Crisp Bar	46	low	1 bar
Nutrisystem® White Chocolate Chunk Cookie	49	low	1 cookie
Nutrisystem® Zesty Herb Snack Mix	54	low	1 package
Optifast VLCD Berry Crunch Bar	25	low	2 oz
Optifast VLCD Cappuccino Flavor Bar	29	low	2 oz
Optifast VLCD Chocolate Bar	20	low	2.5 oz
SlimFast® Meal Options Bar, rich chocolate brownie flavor	64	med	2 oz

@ part of GI symbol program   ★ little or no carbs

HOUSEHOLD MEASURE	CALORIES	FAT (g)	SATURATED FAT (g)	CARBO-HYDRATE (g)	FIBER (g)	SODIUM (mg)
1 bar	160	5	2	25	3	95
1 patty	160	5	4	25	5	30
1 package	100	4	1	14	5	230
1 bar	150	4	3	24	4	150
1 cookie	160	7	3	17	4	65
1 package	120	4	2	16	4	290
1 bar	228	7	2.5	21	5	390
1 bar	226	7	2.5	20	5	390
1 bar	226	7.5	3	13	2	250
1 bar	220	5	4	34	2	170

Subscribe to *GI NEWS* for all the latest – ginews.blogspot.com

GI News is the free, monthly online newsletter from the University of Sydney's Human Nutrition Unit with over 100,000 subscribers worldwide. It's easy to search for topics of interest, and you can post your comments and queries on the site.

Each issue includes:

- The latest research on the glycemic index, carbohydrates, diet, and diabetes along with other hot nutrition topics
- GI Update from Professor Jennie Brand-Miller
- GI Symbol News from Dr. Alan Barclay
- The latest GI values from GI labs in Canada and SUGiRS in Australia
- Recipes from the *GI News* Kitchen, created by dietitian Johanna Burana, *Money Saving Meals* author Diane Temple, and from guest chefs and food writers
- Taste of Health segment by dietitian and author Nicole Senior

www.glycemicindex.com

Search our database for the latest foods tested at the home of the Glycemic Index and discover the answers to the 20 most frequently asked questions about the glycemic index.

- What is the difference between glycemic index (GI) and glycemic load (GL)?

- Should I use GI or GL and does it really matter?

- Do I need to eat only low GI foods at every meal to see a benefit?

- Why do many high-fiber foods still have a high GI value?

- Can I download or can you email me a full list of all GI food values?

- Does the GI increase with serving size? If I eat twice as much, does the GI double?

- If testing continued long enough, wouldn't you expect the areas under the curve to become equal, even for very high and very low GI foods?

- Why doesn't the GI of beef, chicken, fish, tofu, eggs, nuts, seeds, avocados, many fruits (including berries) and vegetables, wine, beer and spirits appear on the GI database?

- Some vegetables appear to have a high GI. Does this mean a person with diabetes should avoid eating them?

- Can you tell me the GI of alcoholic beverages (beer, wine, and spirits)?

- Why does some variability occur in the GI for the same food types?

- Why does pasta have a low GI?

- Most breads and potatoes have a high GI. Does this mean I should never eat them?

- What about flour? If I make my own bread (or dumplings, pancakes, muffins, etc.) which flours, if any, are low GI? What about sprouted grain breads?

- Some high fat foods have a low GI. Doesn't this give a falsely favorable impression of that food?

- Why not just adopt a low carbohydrate diet (like the Atkins diet) to keep my blood glucose levels and weight down?

- Is there a GI Plan for nursing mothers?

- How relevant is the GI for athletes?

- I have recently been diagnosed with celiac disease (gluten sensitivity). It's extremely hard to find both low GI and wheat-free foods. Any suggestions?

- Is a low GI diet suitable for vegetarians?

Where to go for further help

For further information on GI

www.glycemicindex.com

This is the University of Sydney's glycemic index website where you can learn about GI and access the GI database, which includes the most up-to-date listing of the GI of foods that have been published in international scientific journals.

www.gisymbol.com

The Glycemic Index (GI) Symbol Program is a food labeling program with strict nutritional criteria that aims to help people make informed food choices. The site includes a complete listing of foods carrying the GI symbol.

http://ginews.blogspot.com

GI News is the University of Sydney Human Nutrition Unit's official glycemic index monthly newsletter. Subscribing is free.

For further information and advice, we recommend that you contact the following organizations.

American Diabetes Association (ADA)

ADA is the nation's leading nonprofit health organization for people with diabetes in the United States, providing information on diabetes and diabetes prevention, as well as tips and resources for living well with diabetes.

ADA has offices nationwide; to find the office closest to you, call 800-DIABETES (800-342-2383).
www.diabetes.org

American Heart Association

The American Heart Association has offices all around the country. Contact the Heartline at 800-AHA-USA-1 (800-242-8721) for information, or go to their website.
www.americanheart.org

Canadian Diabetes Association

The Canadian Diabetes Association is the national peak consumer health organization for people with diabetes in Canada. The aim of the organization is to promote the health of Canadians through diabetes research, education, service, and advocacy.
800-BANTING (800-226-8464)
www.diabetes.ca

Diabetes Educators

In the United States

American Association of Diabetes Educators (AADE)
200 W. Madison St., Suite 800
Chicago, IL 60606
800-338-3633
www.diabeteseducator.org

In Canada

Canadian Diabetes Educator Certification Board
13909 Hurontario Street
North Suite
Caledon, ON L7C 2C9
905-838-4898
www.cdecb.ca

Dietitians

In the United States
American Dietetic Association
120 South Riverside Plaza, Suite 2000
Chicago, Illinois 60606
800-877-1600
www.eatright.org

In Canada

Dietitians of Canada
480 University Avenue, Suite 604
Toronto, ON M5G 1V2
416-596-0857
www.dieticians.ca

Exercise Specialists

In the United States
American Physical Therapy Association
800-999-APTA (800-999-2782)
www.apta.org and click on "Find a PT"

American Society of Exercise Physiologists

www.asep.org

In Canada

Canadian Physiotherapy Association

955 Green Valley Crescent, Suite 270

Ottawa, ON K2C 3V4

800-387-8679

www.physiotherapy.ca and click on "Find a
Physiotherapist"

Canadian Society for Exercise Physiology

18 Louisa Street, Suite 370

Ottawa, ON K1R 6Y6

Toll-free: 877-651-3755

Tel: 613-234-3775

www.csep.ca

Gluten Intolerance and Celiac Disease

National Institutes of Health Celiac Disease
Awareness Campaign

www.celiac.nih.gov

Celiac Disease Foundation

www.celiac.org

Gluten Intolerance Group
www.gluten.net
www.glutenfree.com

Heart and Stroke Foundation (Canada)
222 Queen Street, Suite 1402
Ottawa, ON K1P 5V9
Call 613-569-4361 to find the Heart and Stroke
Foundation office nearest you.
www.heartandstroke.com

HopeLine (United States)
800-394-HOPE (800-394-4673)
www.thehopeline.com

Juvenile Diabetes Research Foundation International
800-533-CURE (800-533-2873)
www.jdrf.org and click on "Locations"

Kids Help Phone (Canada)
800-668-6868
www.kidshelpphone.ca

Mood Disorder Society of Canada

For anyone suffering from depression and all other
mood disorders, including depression, bipolar
disorders, and anxiety, Mood Disorder Society
provides resources to find help.
304 Stone Road West, Suite 736
Guelph, ON N1G 4W4
519-824-5565
www.mooddisorderscanada.ca

National Alliance on Mental Illness (NAMI) (United States)

NAMI provides information and support for people
living with mental illnesses and their friends and
family.
3803 N. Fairfax Drive, Suite 100
Arlington, VA 22203
Info helpline: 800-950-NAMI (800-950-6264)
www.nami.org

Podiatrists

In the United States

American Podiatric Medical Association
9312 Old Georgetown Road
Bethesda, MD 20814
301-581-9200
www.apma.org

In Canada

Canadian Podiatric Medical Association
#2063, 61 Broadway Boulevard
Sherwood Park, AB T8H 2C1
888-220-3338
www.podiatrycanada.org

Stop Smoking

If you need help to stop smoking, call
United States: 800-QUIT-NOW (800-784-8669)
or visit: smokefree.gov
Canada: 866-225-0709
or visit: Health Canada hc-sc.gc.ca

Acknowledgments

We would like to thank the dedicated GI testing team at SUGiRS—Karola Landry, Kai Lin Ek-Rhodes, Courtney Wright, and Clair de Sousa—and all our cheerful, well-fed, and patient volunteers. We would also like to thank Associate Professor Gareth Denyer for his invaluable help with the GI database and Dr. Alan Barclay from the GI Symbol Program for the sugars and sweeteners information and for thoroughly checking the GI tables for us.

Thank you to dietitian Dr. Kate Marsh, who helped us with the Low GI gluten-free eating section, GI News editor Philippa Sandall, our US editor, Renee Sedliar, and everyone at Hachette Livre Australia who has worked so hard on our behalf, especially Fiona Hazard, Kate Ballard, and Jessica Luca.

Also Available

ISBN: 978-0-7382-1389-7
$16.95

THE LOW GI HANDBOOK

The completely revised and up-dated *New York Times*-bestselling guide to the long-term benefits of low GI eating.

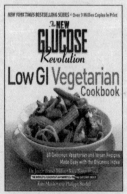

ISBN: 978-1-56924-278-0
$19.95

THE NEW GLUCOSE REVOLUTION LOW GI VEGETARIAN COOKBOOK

The perfect cookbook for vegetarians and vegans looking to eat the right carbs. Features beautiful color photographs and more than 80 recipes low on the glycemic index.

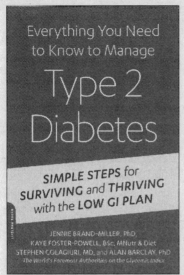

Everything You Need
to Know to Manage

Type 2
Diabetes

SIMPLE STEPS for
SURVIVING and THRIVING
with the LOW GI PLAN

JENNIE BRAND-MILLER, PhD,
KAYE FOSTER-POWELL, BSc, MNutr & Diet
STEPHEN COLAGIURI, MD, and ALAN BARCLAY, PhD
The World's Foremost Authorities on the Glycemic Index

ISBN: 978-0-7382-1847-2
$15.99 / $18.50 Can

EVERYTHING YOU NEED TO KNOW TO MANAGE
TYPE 2 DIABETES

The world's foremost authorities on the glycemic index offer this practical guide to help diabetics of all ages and sizes manage their condition. Revised to focus on prediabetes and type 2, and updated throughout, the handbook offers clear and simple guidelines including what readers should eat and do to reduce body fat, improve insulin sensitivity, strengthen cardiovascular health, and maintain optimal blood glucose levels.

"Dr. Brand-Miller's pioneering research has shown that carbohydrates are not created equal—and everyone having problems with glucose metabolism needs to know the difference."
    Walter Willett, MD, Harvard School of Public Health